Health Care Responsibility

The Older Adult's Guide to Surviving the Health Care System

Raymond Lengel, MSN, CNP, RN

First Edition
HCR Books
North Ridgeville, Ohio

HEALTH CARE RESPONSIBILITY
THE OLDER ADULT'S GUIDE TO SURVIVING THE HEALTH CARE SYSTEM
BY RAYMOND LENGEL

ISBN 1-57087-697-5

Library of Congress Control Number: 2006938446

Cover Design by SHS Design

Lengel, Raymond, 1972-

Health Care Responsibility: The Older Adult's Guide to Surviving the Health Care System/ Raymond Lengel. First Edition

Includes bibliographical references (p.) and index.

1.   Health Care—Popular works

2.   Older Adults—Popular

Published by: HCR Books
P.O. Box 39655
North Ridgeville, OH 44039

Web site: http://www.hcrbooks.com

Printed in the United States of America

CONTENTS

Section 5: Appendixes

Appendix A—Essential Forms

Appendix B—Encounter Forms

ABOUT THE AUTHOR

Raymond Lengel, a certified family nurse practitioner, has worked exclusively in the field of geriatrics for the last four years. In addition to being a certified nurse practitioner, he is a registered nurse with the state of Ohio.

Five years of his professional career involved helping older adults manage chronic diseases including diabetes, lung disease, heart disease, high cholesterol, high blood pressure, osteoporosis, arthritis, and stroke. He has helped patients manage chronic disease through exercise, nutrition, and education and helped them work with their doctor.

Initially, Raymond received a bachelor of science degree in exercise science from the Ohio State University. He wanted to help people with chronic disease and attained a bachelor of science degree in nursing from the Allen College of Nursing in Waterloo, Iowa. After working for a number of years as an exercise physiologist/registered nurse, he enrolled at Otterbein College in Westerville, Ohio, and got a master of science degree in nursing.

His writing career includes a number of online continuing education courses developed for nurses on Parkinson's disease, low-carbohydrate diets, and high blood pressure. His article, "Right to Die," detailing the failing health and eventual death of his first nursing home patient was published in the magazine *Long Term Care Interface*.

Raymond has also presented a number of lectures on a multitude of health care topics including influenza, cardiac risk reduction, stress management, exercise, and nutrition.

ACKNOWLEDGEMENTS

There are a handful of people responsible for helping me write and publish this book. I would like to extend a grateful thanks to my editor Melanie Rigby. I would also like to thank the many individuals and companies responsible for helping me put together the book including my cover designer and my printer, Professional Press.

Most of all I would like to thank my family, Liz, Luke, Anna and Sam for having patience with me as I spent many hours on the process of writing and publishing the book.

DISCLAIMER

This book is designed to provide basic information about the health care system and the patient's role in helping to manage his or her own health. It is sold with the understanding that each individual is unique and the book cannot provide individual advice to any one person.

This book is meant to complement and enhance your interaction with the health care system, not to serve as an alternative to medical advice or care. Utilize the system presented in this book, but be sure to work with your doctor. Your doctor is the best source of health care information for you and the unique set of conditions that are present in your body.

The author has extended every effort to make sure this book is complete and as accurate as possible. Medicine is an evolving field and ongoing research may raise some questions about some of the data in the book. There may be mistakes, both in content and typographical. The book should be used as a general guide and not as the final source for your health care information. Information is current only up to the printing date.

The goal of this book is to educate and entertain. The author and publisher will not have liability or responsibility to any person or entity to any loss or damage to have be caused by information in this book

If you do not wish to be bound by the above, you may return this book to the publisher for a refund.

SECTION 1

INTRODUCTION: THE IMPORTANCE OF HEALTH CARE RESPONSIBILITY

CHAPTER 1

Personal Health Care Responsibility

American health care faces major problems such as the increasing number of older adults and fewer providers to care for them. No easy fix exists; to ensure good health care, you must assume health care responsibility. Many resources are available, and we must know how to best utilize them. By the end of the book, the reader will be equipped with the knowledge to assume health care responsibility.

The goal of this book is to provide a framework for partnering with the health care system. Doctors do not have all of the answers; they require the help of their patients. The information that you provide your doctor assures great health care.

Section 1: Introduction: The Importance of Health Care Responsibility

The first section of this book outlines some of the problems with the health care system. It is important to have an understanding of these problems so you can combat them. In order to avoid bad medical care, each individual must take control of each health care encounter. This goes against the grain of the paternalistic view of medicine in which it is assumed that doctor knows best. Today's health care system is not set up for such a view. Each individual needs to be his or her own advocate. A passive voice will not suffice; being a proactive member of your health care team is the only way to avoid disaster.

The second chapter looks at problems with the health care system and why they are dangerous for the individual patient. This chapter outlines why advances in the health care system have contributed to its downfall. It describes why health care is so expensive, including doctors who practice defensive medicine, health care fragmentation, problems with preventative health care, insurance companies, the costs of drugs, and greed. The chapter also looks at problems with certain sections of the system, including nursing homes, hospitals, and doctors' offices.

Most doctors do not have the time to give you the health care that you deserve. If you can live with suboptimal care, then just go along with the flow. Otherwise, you need to take control. It is your body and you have to live with the outcomes of your health care.

The majority of health care providers are caring individuals who want to give you the best care that they can. Nonetheless, no one is more concerned with your personal health than you are. Each individual must take into account that providers are very busy and often take short cuts just to get through the day. It is critical that consumers are knowledgeable, prepared and organized when interacting in the health care system.

The third chapter gives an overview of the aging process. It explains why the health care system is not ready for the growing aging population. The effect aging has on the overall health of an individual, including how aging can significantly decrease quality of life and increase functional impairment, is discussed.

Section 2: Surviving the Health Care System

The second section provides tips to help patients communicate more effectively within the health care system. Americans are cared for in settings including doctors' offices, hospitals, urgent care clinics, emergency rooms, and nursing homes. Effective communication involves talking not only to your doctor, but also to the staff.

Medicine is big business that is driven by money, and too often patient care is a secondary goal. Some physicians see six to eight patients an hour. The result is poor quality health care.

Communication is an essential skill to get the best care possible. It requires skill to optimize time with the doctor to transmit and extract essential information. Communication is a challenging skill to master; knowledge and preparation are key components. This section provides a method and forms for transmitting essential information to your health care provider.

As part of the focus on communication skills, chapters 5 and 6 outline the risks in hospitals and nursing homes and share strategies to improve the quality of your care in these venues.

Medications have improved health care quality, but they are not without risk. Chapter 7 looks at ways to assure your medication regime is appropriate. It explains why patients are on so many medications and why this is such a big concern. It addresses the major concerns with medications including side effects, drug interactions, adverse drug reactions, compliance with medication prescriptions, over-the-counter drugs, and overexposure to drugs.

SECTION 3: HEALTH PROMOTION AND DISEASE PREVENTION

Preventative health care incorporates a broad variety of activities to prevent problems before they occur or catch them before they do too much damage to the body. The three main components to preventative health care include: healthy lifestyle, health screenings, and immunizations. Exercising, establishing good nutrition habits, stopping or not starting smoking, minimizing alcohol intake, receiving recommended immunizations, and having recommended health screenings are examples.

General goals of preventative health care are to decrease premature death and increase quality of life. Each individual also has specific goals. Someone who is healthy uses preventative medicine to stay healthy, while individuals with multiple chronic diseases use preventative medicine to prevent further disability and deterioration.

The American health care system misses many opportunities for preventative medicine. Do not assume that your doctor will remember to discuss, recommend, or provide all the necessary measures. Most doctors simply have too many patients and not enough time to do a complete job at preventative medicine. Patients need to take responsibility. Many aspects of preventative medicine are completely up to the individual while others require collaboration between patient and the health care provider.

Chapter 8 provides guidelines to help you track your preventative health care. The chapter concludes with an example of how preventative medicine can help maximize quality and quantity of life. Worksheets are provided to help you track recommended screenings, exams, immunizations, blood tests, counseling, and diagnostic tests.

Not exercising can kill you. Physical inactivity is responsible for hundreds of thousands of deaths each year. In addition, exercise helps you maintain a high quality of life. The aging body goes through numerous changes that lead to disability, and rates of disability are increased in inactive individuals.

The ability to perform tasks once taken for granted often becomes tremendously difficult with age. The decrease in strength and endurance can render the older adult less able to handle routine tasks of daily living. For example, bringing the groceries in from the car is a simple task that with aging becomes exceedingly difficult. Individuals who regularly exercise are more likely to maintain function and continue doing such tasks without difficulty.

Good nutrition is an essential step in preserving good health. A healthy diet maintains a healthy body weight, prevents disease, and minimizes the effects of established disease. There is much confusion about what constitutes good nutrition. This chapter highlights research findings to help clarify specific measures that readers can take to improve nutrition.

Chapter 9 defines exercise and provides guidelines to help the reader comply with national recommendations to maximize health. The chapter includes a list of benefits and risks of exercise. It helps the reader understand how much, how hard, how long, and how frequently to exercise. It looks at three types of exercise: aerobic exercise, strength training, and stretching.

Chapter 10 explores the benefits of healthy eating and the risks of not eating healthy. The topics discussed include obesity, weight loss, specific vitamins and minerals, and the relationship of nutrition and disease. The focus of this chapter is to empower the older adult with the knowledge of how to maximize health through nutrition.

This section gives an overview of exercise and nutrition and provides tips to improve your diet and exercise habits. It also provides questions to discuss with your health care provider to assure you are eating and exercising properly.

SECTION 4: PUTTING IT ALL TOGETHER

Obtaining a proper medical history is one of the most time-consuming jobs of a health care provider. Older Americans have complex medical histories, and getting a good medical history could be the difference between life and death. Being prepared for every health care encounter is an essential step in transmitting a complete and concise medical history. Older Americans are at high risk for falling through the cracks and suffering from complications of a compromised health care system. Reporting an accurate medical history can make the difference.

This section provides a format to organize your health care information and report it to your provider. It outlines a system using the concepts described in this book to help you obtain optimal health. *The system is broken down into seven steps to allow you to simply organize and communicate your health care information.* It is a simple system, but it does take time and preparation. It reviews how to maintain your personal health record and supplies forms to track your health. It gives an overview of how to transmit proper information to your health care provider in different situations.

Personal health care responsibility—when each individual assumes responsibility for his or her health—can alleviate many of the problems with the current system. This does not mean you will be making your own diagnosis or prescribing your own treatment. But you will be organizing your information to help the provider give you optimal care.

APPENDIXES

The first appendix has a listing of essential forms that all readers should fill out as part of his or her personal medical record.

The second appendix includes forms to prepare and communicate vital information for annual doctor visits, sick visits, and follow-up visits. Completion of hospital and nursing home communication forms, referral forms, and emergency room forms is discussed.

HOW A PERSONAL HEALTH CARE RECORD CAN HELP

After moving in with her son, an eighty-year-old woman goes to a new primary care physician for a complete history and physical exam. She is diagnosed with diabetes and high blood pressure and is started on a medicine to control her blood pressure called an angiotensin-converting enzyme inhibitor and is told to follow up in one week with the diabetes educator and in two weeks with the doctor.

Ten days later, the primary care physician receives a call from the emergency room explaining that his new patient is in the emergency room with an irregular heart rate and a high potassium level. He calls the woman's daughter, with whom she lived previously, to get more details on the patient's history. He finds out that the patient has a much more extensive medical history than she indicated during her initial appointment. In fact, he determines that she only reported about one-half of the medical information that he needed to treat her adequately.

This situation is not solely the fault of the patient or the doctor. Older patients have complicated medical histories, and many patients are unable to recall pertinent details during the pressure of an office visit. In addition, doctors often do not take or have the time to ask the proper questions.

The patient's most significant omission was the diagnosis of renal artery stenosis, which was diagnosed five years earlier. In renal artery stenosis, the arteries to the kidneys are narrowed and the use of certain blood pressure medications such as angiotensin-converting enzyme inhibitors or angiotensin receptor blockers can lead to serious side effects.

This situation could have been prevented with the accurate reporting of a complete medical history. Unfortunately, this is not an uncommon occurrence. Iatrogenic disease, disease caused by medical treatment, is commonplace in health care. The use of a preplanned medical record form can greatly improve the ability to transmit information to the provider and prevent health care issues.

A TYPICAL PATIENT

Teri is a sixty-two-year-old female who lives with her husband. She was diagnosed with high blood pressure when she was thirty-two. She thinks she has had abnormal cholesterol at some point in her life, but is unable to recall the details. She has had no surgical procedures and has been hospitalized only with the births of her two children. Her medications include two pills for her blood pressure and an aspirin. She recently quit smoking but smoked one pack of cigarettes a day for thirty years. She drinks alcohol occasionally.

Teri's doctor recently retired, so she goes to a new doctor. The medical record obtained from her previous doctor is incomplete and illegible. She has vague complaints of feeling tired, coughing more over the year, and having dry skin.

SCENARIO #1

Teri visits her new doctor who generously spends twenty minutes asking questions, reviewing her medical history, and performing a physical exam. The first ten minutes of the visit involves the doctor getting a medical history from her. Obtaining a medical history takes a significant amount of time, especially with patients who are older and those who have complicated histories.

During the interview, Teri reports that she is very healthy. She reports that she had a bunch of tests to check her cholesterol, thyroid, kidneys, heart, and lungs within the last year and they did not reveal any problems. She is unable to provide specifics or produce any hard copies of the tests.

The doctor examines Teri for the next five minutes. Then, during the last five minutes of the appointment, the doctor explains his findings and gives some general advice. He concludes by giving Teri a prescription for multiple blood tests and a chest X-ray. The next appointment to review the results of the tests is scheduled for three weeks later.

The next appointment lasts only ten minutes and focuses on reviewing her multiple medical tests. The doctor comes into the appointment, reads the results, answers a few misplaced questions from Teri, and is out the door. Teri is left with a prescription for more medical tests, a prescription for a different blood pressure pill, another follow-up appointment in two weeks, and many unanswered questions.

Teri returns to the doctor's office for follow-up on her next battery of blood tests. It is determined that she has diabetes, an underactive thyroid, and poorly controlled cholesterol. The doctor adds medication for these conditions. Teri leaves the appointment very confused. She has multiple unanswered questions about her health and the new medicines. She also continues to cough and is having a difficult time breathing with exercise.

Scenario #2

Teri meets with her new doctor and presents him a detailed medical history (the personal health record in Chapter 11). In addition, she provides him with a detailed report of her symptoms on a prepared medical form (the annual/initial visit form in Chapter 4). She also presents a list of questions that she is most concerned about. Teri spent thirty minutes gathering information and preparing a list of questions before the appointment.

The doctor is able to focus more of his attention on Teri's concerns because he does not have to work as hard at extracting necessary medical information. Instead of running multiple medical tests, he is able to focus tests based on her history and the results of previous tests.

Because of the accurate reporting of her history, Teri had more specific blood tests and a lung function test, which resulted in a prompt and accurate diagnosis. She was diagnosed with chronic obstructive lung disease, hypothyroidism, high cholesterol, and diabetes. Treatment was initiated for each of these conditions on the next visit, which was scheduled one week after the results of the laboratory analysis returned.

In the first scenario, important tests were not done. Health care providers are reluctant to order every test in the book on patients with vague complaints. While some providers will order a battery of diagnostic tests, this is financially irresponsible and medically unadvisable.

Not only will running multiple lab tests on each patient be expensive, it is likely to result in many false-positive results. False positives show an individual having a specific disease or condition, but the results are wrong. False-positives result in more testing, which will result in more discomfort and possible complications for the patient. The more tests that are run, the more at risk a patient is. In addition, this has the potential to cost the medical system billions of dollars a year.

In the first scenario, the doctor erred on the side of doing fewer medical tests. It took more time to diagnose Teri's problems. Teri reported that she had tests that were normal last year. Under the pressure of a time-limited office visit, Teri was unable to recall the exact details or dates of what her previous doctor said two years ago, not one year ago as she reported.

An accurate look at the patient's previous medical history revealed that she had mildly elevated blood sugar levels and a borderline thyroid test two years ago. The lung test that was done was a chest X-ray, which demonstrated possible changes consistent with lung disease. At the time Teri was not having any symptoms, so no treatment for her lungs was started.

With this poor reporting of her medical history, the doctor was unable to diagnose and treat her symptoms promptly. While no serious consequences occurred, the patient had diagnoses delayed and was inconvenienced with multiple unnecessary diagnostic tests, blood work, and doctor visits. It also costs the health care system much more money to perform this battery of tests.

The current healthcare system makes it impossible for providers to have unlimited access to previous medical records. The electronic medical record will make it easier in the future, but that system is not in place now.

It may be thought that the doctor in the first scenario was incompetent and did not do an adequate job in diagnosing the patient's problems, but this is not the case. Teri did not reveal any history of thyroid dysfunction or diabetes. If she had, blood tests that are more specific would have been run instead of basic screening protocols. She reported a normal chest X-ray when her X-ray in fact had been abnormal. If the new doctor had been aware of the abnormal chest X-ray, he would have ordered a repeat X-ray and a test to determine if she had any damage to her lungs. This would have shored up a diagnosis of chronic obstructive lung disease and would have helped explain Teri's increased coughing and shortness of breath on exertion. Having hard copies of diagnostic tests and blood work are a key component to getting good health care. A patient's recollection of the interpretations is often different from the actual test result.

In the second scenario, the doctor noticed that Teri's previous thyroid levels were very slightly elevated, though not enough to warrant treatment. He also noticed that Teri's father had diabetes and noted a very minimal increase in her blood sugar on the previous lab draw. Based on this, the doctor ordered a more specific test for diabetes and thyroid disease. He also ordered a complete cholesterol panel, which revealed cholesterol readings greater than recommended in patients with diabetes.

Taking care of patients is an extremely challenging job, and doctors are unable to care for their patients if they do not get an adequate history. While it is a shared responsibility between doctor and patient, the main responsibility for a good history falls on the patient. Most doctors will dedicate thirty minutes to seeing a new patient, but the actual face-to-face time is usually closer to twenty minutes. It is almost impossible to get a complete history on a patient over the age of fifty who has had multiple medical encounters and numerous problems. The older patient has generally seen many different providers, had many tests, and has been on multiple medications. For these reasons it is essential that you take personal health care responsibility and report your medical history as succinctly and completely as possible.

When visiting with a doctor, especially for the first time, patients have a tendency to get nervous and do a poor job transmitting information. This is a major problem, because this is the most important thing that can be done during the visit. If you take responsibility for your health, you will greatly enhance your odds to get the best health care possible.

Your Health Is Your Responsibility

Doctors are not solely responsible for making the final health care decisions; it is a team effort. You need to depend on your doctor's expertise and listen to recommendations, but do not let the doctor dictate the care.

The average health care appointment is about ten to fifteen minutes. It important that you maximize the time. Come into your appointment organized: have a written copy of your medical history, record your problem before you get there, and have questions prepared for the doctor.

Learning to communicate with the health care system is the point of this book. Improved communication with the system is a central step to improving health.

This book guides you through the process of setting up your personal health record. It will help you gather all the vital information a provider needs. By the end of the book, you will be able to:

- Transmit your complete and concise medical history to any provider.

- Track your preventative health care, including knowing what testing you need.

- Understand how to communicate with your provider.

- Feel confident that you are a partner in managing your health.

CHAPTER 2

AMERICA'S HEALTH CARE SYSTEM: THE PROBLEMS

The World Health Organization reports that the United States has the thirty-seventh best health care system in the world.[1] The U.S. system is fraught with problems and its patient satisfaction is rated among the worst in the world. In the developed world, the United States is at the bottom of the list for infant mortality and life expectancy.

Health care is not the same as it was fifty years ago. Medical science has made tremendous advances in the treatment of heart disease, cancer, infectious diseases, and diabetes, just to name a few, but these advances have come at a cost. The personal touch of medicine has been lost.

THE UNITED STATES HAS EXPENSIVE HEALTH CARE

Health care in America is the most expensive in the world. In 2004, the United States spent $6,280 in per capita health expenditures, over 50 percent more than any other country.[2] Factors include the cost of medications, top-rate medical technologies, the extensive use of diagnostic tests, salaries of doctors and hospital administrators, government regulations, and increasing life expectancy.

Medications are expensive to develop, and drug companies want to turn a profit. Incorporated into the price of a medication are many things above and beyond the drug itself. Medications must cover the costs of producing new compounds that become established drugs. The cost of compounds that scientists work on for years but that do not become drugs also is included. New medications need to go through a rigorous and long approval process.

Marketing—including commercials, drug representative salaries, and perks to doctors such as pens, continuing education courses, and meals—also are included. And, drug companies must turn a profit to keep their stockholders happy and to make sure that the company continues to have money to develop new drugs for the future.

Similarly, the development of top medical technologies is expensive. Medical technologies can make tremendous improvements in patient care and outcomes, but they place a financial burden on the health care system. A single MRI scanner can cost over one million dollars and a single scan costs the patient or insurance company about one thousand dollars.

The reliance on expensive diagnostic procedures defines the American health care system and contributes to the increased health care costs. For example, chest X-rays are commonly performed on patients with coughs. While many times this is a necessary diagnostic exam to rule in pneumonia or a flare of congestive heart failure, the test is often ordered when it is not necessary. Multiple reasons—including doctors who don't spend adequate time performing a history and physical exam, fear of litigation, and patient demand—account for the overreliance on diagnostic tests. A complete history and physical exam can sometimes replace the need for diagnostic tests, but many providers feel more comfortable ordering a test rather than spending the time to perform a good history and physical exam.

In addition to the direct cost, many tests discover abnormalities that turn out to be a false. To determine the significance of the abnormalities, the physician needs to run more tests and sometimes initiates treatment.

Doing unnecessary tests based on the results of these false positives contributes to not only increased cost, but also to increased risk for the patient. Many tests can lead to complications that not only mean more cost but also may harm or kill the patient. Today's system focuses more on diagnostic tests than on clinician knowledge not only because doctors are more comfortable with this approach but also because it reimburses better. Procedures are grossly overreimbursed by insurance companies, and the financial responsibilities are removed from the doctor and patient.

Defensive medicine is another factor driving up the cost of medical care. The litigious society that we live in makes it necessary for doctors to cover all of their bases. Delay in diagnosis is a common reason physicians are sued. Because of this, doctors are more prone to order expensive tests to rule out any possibility that a diagnosis can be missed. The practice of defensive medicine costs the American medical system billions of dollars a year.

Malpractice also is driving up costs. Medical fees are higher partly in response to doctors paying higher malpractice premiums. Lawsuits are on the rise for a number of reasons such as unrealistic patient expectations, failure to inform patients of all possible outcomes, and the predatory efforts of lawyers. Lawsuits in health care are necessary to keep doctors practicing safely, but there are many frivolous lawsuits.

Doctor's salaries are increasing, especially specialty doctors such as cardiologists and gastroenterologists. An oversupply of specialists contributes to the rising health care costs. These specialists are eager and enthusiastic to carry out expensive procedures because they result in good payments.

There are other reasons for higher costs. Health care systems are spending more on advertising as they compete for patients. Large hospitals employ many administrators with salaries topping a hundred thousand dollars. Insurance plans and government regulations increase the amount of paperwork and administrative costs.

The use of the emergency room as a primary care service is costly. Emergency room physicians do not know the patients and are more prone to order expensive tests and treatments.

Health care costs increase for older patients, who have more diseases that are chronic. This translates into increased doctor visits, hospitalizations, medications, and treatments.

GREED

Greed has inundated the health care system. Doctors seeing six to eight patients an hour have replaced the old image of Dr. Marcus Welby sitting down and spending thirty minutes with each patient. Economic incentives are built into our current medical system, and the American medical system is more of a business model than a caring model.

The business aspect of the medical system is disturbing. Doctors are often limited partners in the hospitals or clinics where they work so that they can help keep a financial eye on the system. Administrators are offered lofty bonuses to turn a profit. Methods used to make a profit often involve cutting staffers who are directly responsible for patient care. This creates more stress and decreases the quality of care.

Fewer primary care doctors practice today. Primary care doctors—family practice physicians, internists, general practitioners, and geriatricians—are responsible for handling basic health care concerns. They are essential gatekeepers to controlling health care costs. Due to the lower reimbursement to primary care providers, many physicians are going into specialty practice. The average specialist commands a salary of one hundred thousand dollars a year more than the average primary care doctor.

Doctors want to be rewarded financially for the years of hard work they put into obtaining their degree. Medicine is not as lucrative as it used to be due to decreased reimbursement and increased malpractice premiums. Working within a managed care setting, primary care doctors have to see more patients just to break even.

FRAGMENTATION

Information does not always follow patients. There is no one place that knows all about your health. Fragmented health services are largely responsible for health care information not being in one place. Fragmentation is the use of multiple medical specialists or medical systems to care for one individual. One doctor caring for all of your medical needs is not the norm in today's health care setting. Fragmentation of health care is one by-product of the health care monster in America. Fragmentation leads to duplicate medications and services, which is not only costly, but also potentially harmful or deadly.

An individual with diabetes, heart failure, prostate cancer, and depression could be seeing an endocrinologist (doctor for diabetes), cardiologist (heart doctor), urologist (doctor of the urinary system), oncologist (cancer doctor), psychiatrist, and a primary care doctor. With this many doctors treating the patient, there is a risk of duplication of services, such as two doctors doing the same test or two different doctors prescribing similar or duplicate medications, and of too few tests being run because one doctor assumes the other is doing it. Poor communication between the specialists is commonplace. It is critical that each health care consumer monitor medicines to assure there are no duplications or drugs that interact with one another. It is also essential that each doctor knows which medications each of his patients is on.

Medical specialists are very valuable. With the plethora of research published every month, keeping up to date is not possible for any one doctor. There are over four thousand biomedical journals and over five hundred new medicines or new uses for old drugs per year. Many general physicians worry about their ability to keep up with all of the new information.

While specialists are great resources, caution must be instituted. Providing continuity in the health care system falls on the shoulder of each consumer. The first step is to communicate effectively. The use of the medical record system outlined in this book is an important step in health care responsibility.

Primary care doctors often take care of their own patients in the hospital, but this takes away from their office practice. Consequently, many consult hospitalists, those who specialize in hospital patient care. While hospitalists do a good job, they are typically not familiar with their patients' medical histories. When being cared for by a hospitalist, the use of the personal medical system is critical. It may mean the difference between life and death.

DOCTOR APPOINTMENTS

Doctor appointments fall below the expectation of many patients. The average office visit is approximately ten minutes, and many patients would argue the average visit is much less than this. These ten minutes include reviewing the chart, talking to the patient, examining the patient, charting, answering questions, filling out forms, and giving out prescriptions. The physician is not able to spend adequate time with the patient.

Many patients complain about long waits. Many physicians require an initial visit so that a complete history and physical exam can be performed before the patient is seen for urgent problems. The wait for this initial, more time-consuming appointment can be one to two months. The doctor's office will not see an acutely ill patient unless this initial visit has been carried out.

Insurance Companies

Over forty-five million Americans are without health insurance. Even with insurance, deductibles and copays can add up to tens of thousands of dollars per year. While insurance is necessary, it does limit the care many people receive. Insurance companies are out to make a profit; consequently, they put limits on what medical personnel can do to care for patients. Most insurance companies limit hospital stays and determine which medicines and services patients can receive and even which doctors they can see.

Insurance brokers are highly motivated by high commission rates. Caring for the patient's medical needs are often not the top priority. Insurance company administrators who often do not have a medical background are making medical decisions. Insurance companies often preclude potential clients based on preexisting conditions.

Managed care companies have changed the way that medicine is practiced. Doctors are often very frustrated at being limited in the testing they can perform because of reimbursement issues. The goal of managed care is to keep costs down by focusing on preventative services such as immunization and health screenings. While managed care saves money, there are many justified concerns with the system. Physicians working for the system have less control over what can be ordered. Extensive paperwork is often involved in getting certain procedures and referrals approved.

Capitation is a system that saves a lot of money. It involves giving the primary care provider a set amount of money for each patient in the health care plan. Spending more than a set amount of money on a patient counts against the provider's salary. Spending less than the set amount results in a credit. Under this system, there is an incentive to control costs and limit the amount of care each patient receives. This forces the primary care provider to heavily consider the cost when ordering a test. This reduces the number of expensive tests or procedures ordered. This system brings out a new type of greed: the doctor and health care administrator withholding care to turn a profit.

Debt from health care is a common cause of bankruptcy. The Institute of Medicine showed that approximately eighteen thousand people die each year because of no insurance.[3] This happens because people may wait to obtain health care until the last minute because they are afraid they can't pay for it. This can occur even with patients with adequate health insurance due to high copays and deductibles.

Overutilization also causes insurance companies to increase copays and deductibles. Many doctors refuse Medicare and Medicaid if they can get enough patients on other insurance plans.

NURSING HOMES

Almost 1.9 million individuals were living in nursing homes in 2000. There is a residence rate of nursing home beds of over 87 percent.[4]

Patients are often admitted to nursing homes after hospitalization that left them unable to care for themselves. Some individuals are in nursing homes for short-term rehabilitative stays, but many patients are there long term.

Nursing home patients are usually assigned doctors who are unfamiliar with their medical history. These are medically complex patients, and knowledge of their medical histories is of great value. Still, rarely does one member of the team caring for the patient have a full understanding of the events that the person has gone through in the last number of weeks or years.

Nursing home patients are unstable and need diligent monitoring. The doctor needs to have an understanding of the patient's history, and someone needs to transmit the information to the nursing home staff.

HOSPITALS

Hospitals are the place to be when you need intense medical care. But hospital care also is laced with complications, and an argument can be made that the hospital is not necessarily the best place for sick patients. Iatrogenic disease—disease caused by medical care—runs rampant in hospital. Some common factors leading to iatrogenic disease include blood transfusions, biopsies, endoscopies, the introduction of new drugs, and surgery. It is hard to get through a hospital stay without the introduction of one of these procedures.

Infection is a common iatrogenic disease. The number of infections acquired in the hospital top two million a year and adds days and thousands of dollars to the typical stay. The most common infections acquired in the hospital include urinary tract infections, pneumonia, surgical site infections, and primary blood stream infections. The scariest part of the saga is that many of the nosicomial (hospital-acquired) infections are resistant to many of the antibiotics currently available.

New medications commonly are added into the patient's medical treatment during a hospital stay, and these new drugs have the potential for an adverse drug reaction. Adverse drug reactions, described more in a later chapter, account for over a hundred thousand deaths each year.[5]

Hospital care often is not as good as it could be. Many hospitals are cutting staff members or replacing them with less qualified—and cheaper—replacements. In an effort to improve the bottom line, medical assistants are replacing registered nurses. Registered nurses have at least two, and often four, years of training while medical aides may have only had a week of training.

Medical errors occur at an alarming rate. The Institute of Medicine reported that 44,000 to 98,000 people die each year in the hospital due to medical errors.[6] Many of these errors are covered up and death is written off to the underlying disease process.

PREVENTATIVE HEALTH CARE

The health care system of the United States focuses more on curative care than preventative care. More money can be made curing and treating disease than preventing disease. Preventative medicine can prevent disease from occurring or result in diagnoses before signs and symptoms or complications arise, increasing the chance for recovery. Preventative medicine involves healthy eating, exercise, smoking cessation, decreased alcohol use, injury prevention, the use of diagnostic tests to catch diseases early, and the use of vaccines. Insurance companies pay for some preventative services, but many are not covered.

America has become an obese and sedentary society. We are involved in more spectator sports than participant sports. We have less physical education in schools. We watch television and play videogames instead of exercising.

Lack of exercise is a common predecessor of disease. The implementation of a regular exercise program significantly reduces the risk of many diseases including obesity, which can lead to significant health care problems. Weight loss can provide many health benefits, including increased quality of life, decreased blood pressure, improved cholesterol, and a reduction in diabetes and heart disease.

HOW TO GET THE BEST HEALTH CARE IN THE WORLD

Despite its many problems, many experts would argue that the United States has the best health care system in the world. Many foreign diplomats come to the United States to receive health care. If you know how to take advantage of it, America has the best health care in the world. To get it, you need to be educated, organized, and able to communicate.

Being educated does not mean that you need to have a medical degree or even a high school diploma. It means that you know how to get and transmit critical information. Having a system to organize and communicate your health information will significantly improve health care.

Individuals who ask questions tend to get better health care. Diseases are not universal. Each individual must understand how his or her disease affects him or her personally. It is not enough to read a book about a chronic disease that you have and feel you have a firm understanding of how that disease affects you.

The current capitalistic health care system focuses on profit instead of patient care. This does not mean that you cannot receive great health care in the current system. It does mean that you will have to do more than have a good doctor. You need to take responsibility for your health care. Health care responsibility includes understanding your health and disease states, organizing your health information and communicating it with the system.

CHAPTER 3

Aging America

Sixty-year-old John retires after thirty-five years of teaching high school chemistry. He enjoys his newfound freedom by dining out more frequently and gains twenty pounds. This causes his arthritis to hurt more, and consequently he decreases his activity from power walking thirty minutes four nights a week to riding a stationary bike for fifteen minutes one to two times a week. He also notices increased difficulty breathing when walking, so he discontinues his after-dinner walk with his wife in favor of reading and watching television. Over the next year, his weight remains stable but his muscles begin to shrink. In an attempt to get back on track, he hires a personal trainer who determines that his body fat is 30 percent and he has very poor strength.

Before John starts his exercise program, at his personal trainer's request he visits his doctor, who determines that he has high blood pressure. He puts John on blood pressure medicine and an aspirin. The blood pressure pill makes him feel tired and he puts his exercise program on hold. During the next three months, he suffers a very minor stroke, which leaves him with a slight amount of weakness on his left side.

Feeling better, he resumes exercising and has an extra hard workout at the gym. The next morning, he notices his muscles are extremely sore; while walking down the stairs to get his breakfast, he falls and breaks his right hip. He has surgery and goes through rehabilitation but is still severely limited. His rehabilitation is complicated by a number of infections and illness secondary to his overall poor health. Close to the end of his rehabilitation, he goes back to the doctor with a complaint of a tremor in his right hand. His doctor diagnoses him as having early Parkinson's disease.

He is told by his rehabilitation doctor and physical therapist that he is fully recovered but he does not feel the way he did a year ago. He is unable to walk without a walker. It takes him twice as long to get ready in the morning and to eat a meal. He now suffers from major depression.

America is in crisis. According to the Administration on Aging, the population of individuals over sixty-five is 36.3 million and will rise to 71.5 million by 2030.[1]

The health care system is not ready for the increasing number of geriatric clients, who have special medical needs. The American Geriatrics Society reports that the number of physicians to care for geriatric patients is about 35 percent of what is needed. In addition, less than 1 percent of registered nurses are trained in geriatrics.

Experts have many concerns about how America will handle this boom in population among older adults. Fewer working adults relative to the over sixty-five population will lead to many problems. The working population supports both financially and physically the older population's health care. Will there be enough money to meet the health care and general care needs when the baby boom population hits its peak? Even if there is enough money, will there be enough people to care for them? Will there be enough nursing home beds and hospital beds?

The fast-paced health care system often leaves the older patient behind. Older patients move slower, hear poorly, and take longer to express and recall information. Older patients need to relay their complete medical history, any new problems, and pertinent information about chronic diseases.

Why Is the Older Population Increasing?

The number of older Americans is increasing as baby boomers enter their golden years. Other factors include increased life expectancy, decreased infant death rates, and medical advancement.

The baby boomer generation, people born between 1946 and 1964, is the largest number of people born in the history of America. This increased birth rate was the result of economic prosperity experienced after World War II. This generation comprises 76 million people.

Life expectancy is expected to increase in the developed world from 76 years old to 80 years old. In 2000, the life expectancy for the total population was 77.9 years old.[2] Life expectancy was around 50 in the early 1900s. Sanitation improvements, such as the introduction of sewers, reduced the spread of disease and contributed to the prolonged life expectancy. Medical advances are another large contributor to the increased life expectancy. The infant death rate is currently around five per thousand; in the 1920s, the rate was about seventy per thousand. More infants surviving translates into more people living into their golden years.

Medical advances also have decreased death rates from many acute and chronic illnesses. With the advent of antibiotics and immunizations, incidents of infectious disease, which used to be the leading cause of death, declined. Today, pneumonia/influenza is the only infectious cause of death in the top ten. Chronic conditions such as high blood pressure, diabetes, and heart disease are responsible for the development of the most common causes of death today. The medical community is becoming more skilled at treating these conditions, yet they are still common causes of death and disability. Medicine has made advances in treatment of heart disease and stroke, but cancer death rates have remained stable. If we are to be successful in extending life expectancy, we are going to need to control these chronic conditions.

Why should we be so concerned with the aging population? The older people are, the more likely they are to die. Older age also puts you at risk for disease and a poor quality of life. Aging is associated with decreased function and frailty. These concerns can be minimized by good health care. That decision is up to each individual. Do you want to take charge of your health care, or do you want to sit idly by and let your health deteriorate and let the medical system walk all over you?

AGING AND YOUR BODY

At some point, which is different for every individual and every body system, organs and tissues in the human body deteriorate. The likelihood of developing disease increases as people age. This does not mean that aging will predictably result in disease, but there is increased risk of disease as the body ages. A fine line exists between normal changes of aging and disease processes. For example, as one ages it is normal to have a decline in your mental processing, but full-blown

Alzheimer's disease is a pathological process and not normal. Healthy aging should be a goal for every individual. This is a challenging venture, but can be accomplished with health care responsibility.

Many of the consequences of aging are a result of unhealthy lifestyles. The six most common causes of death—heart disease, cancer, stroke, chronic lung disease, pneumonia/influenza, and diabetes—are strongly related to lifestyle practices. Health care responsibility involves living a healthy lifestyle: specifically, meaning exercise, good nutrition and partnering with the system to manage your well-being.

Aging Changes

Individuals and body systems age differently, but some changes are universal. It is difficult to draw the line between normal aging and disease states. Common changes associated with aging are listed below.

EYES: Although many changes in the eye are related to disease, some are an inevitable consequence of aging. In the fifth decade, people typically have increasing difficulty seeing objects that are closer than two feet. This leads to difficulty in reading and the reliance on glasses for reading. The lens becomes more yellow and opaque, which affects color and depth perception. The ability of the eye to accommodate is compromised, which means a more difficult time changing the focus of vision from near to far. The incidence of black specks, known as floaters, floating across the visual field is more common as we age. Individuals are more sensitive to glare.

The pupil, which is the black part in the center of the eye and is responsible for allowing light into the back of the eye, goes through multiple changes during the aging process. It narrows, which means that the older individual needs more light to see and has more difficulty going from light to dark environments and vice versa. The pupil becomes less responsive to light, resulting in more sensitivity to light.

EARS: Hearing loss associated with aging is usually bilateral and affects high tones first. Exposure to loud noise over a lifetime is partly responsible for the decreased hearing. Tinnitus, better known as a ringing in the ears, affects 25 percent of the population over sixty-five. Hearing loss is the most common cause of tinnitus, but it can be caused by excessive earwax, fluid in the ear, Meniere's disease, or a tumor.

Earwax, also known as cerumen, tends to accumulate during the aging process. The body is typically able to self-clean the ear. As one ages, earwax becomes drier and has a tendency to stick to the canal, resulting in clumping. Excessive earwax is commonly associated with hearing changes.

SKIN: The aging process is associated with drier, thinner, less elastic, and more wrinkled skin. The ability to sense is also compromised due to a decrease in the number of nerve endings. This leads to an increased risk of burns. Exposure to the sun over the years leads to increased wrinkling and a compromised protective response to sun damage. Long-term sun exposure combined with genetic factors increases the risk of different types of skin cancers.

MUSCULOSKELETAL SYSTEM: Bones thin as one ages, which puts people at increased risk for broken bones. A decrease in sex hormones contributes to the loss of bone strength. While bones lose strength in both sexes, females are much more likely to develop significant bone loss. Height is commonly lost as one ages due to the narrowing of spaces between the vertebrae and compression of the spinal column. Other issues lead to a decrease in bone mass such as decreased activity, cigarette smoking, high thyroid levels, excessive alcohol intake, and certain medications.

The center of the bones, called the marrow, is responsible for producing blood cells. With age, the bone marrow produces fewer blood cells. The red blood cells are important to carry oxygen to the rest of the body. With the decreased production of red blood cells, the body's ability to get oxygen to the cells is decreased, contributing to fatigue.

Muscle mass and strength also diminish. The lining of the joints, known as cartilage, tends to shrink as we age due to wear and tear. Decreased cartilage and fluid in the joints are contributing factors to arthritis.

Heart/Vascular System: A healthy heart functions well into old age, but many subtle changes occur. Heart function is partly affected by how active an individual is throughout his or her life. It is difficult to separate the normal aging processes, the effects of disease, and the effects that decreased physical activity have on the heart.

The aging process results in the heart becoming stiffer and filling with blood more slowly. This leads to a common condition, especially common in older women, called diastolic heart failure. The blood vessel walls become stiffer and less responsive to changes in the amount of blood pumped through them, which leads to an increased frequency of high blood pressure. The nerves in the heart do not function as well, which results in a higher incidence of rhythm disturbances.

Coronary heart disease is much more common in the older population than the younger. The accumulation of plaque (a fatty substance that blocks the vessels) in the arteries around the heart occurs over time. Other factors such as, exposure to cigarette smoke, abnormal cholesterol levels, high blood pressure, and the presence of diabetes increase the risk of plaque formation. Exposure to all of these factors increases over the years and therefore the older one becomes, the more likely he or she is to have heart disease.

Lungs: The healthy lung functions well throughout life. Changes in the lung system, especially in smokers, make breathing more difficult. Changes associated with aging include a weakened diaphragm, a weaker cough, and less oxygen being absorbed into the body. The lung and chest wall stiffen with the aging process. The number of breathing sacs—known as alveoli—decreases with age. Alveoli are responsible for transferring oxygen and waste products between the lungs and the blood.

The breathing system gradually declines with age, but the process is sped up when disease is present. A lifetime of exposure to toxins, with cigarettes being the most prevalent, along with the aging process results in a declining lung function.

DIGESTIVE SYSTEM: The ability to taste food decreases, contributing to weight loss in the older population. Due to the valves in the digestive tract not working as efficiently as they once did, the older patient is more like to suffer from heartburn. The stomach lining is much more likely to incur damage, increasing the propensity for ulcers. The stomach is less elastic and empties more slowly. Food byproducts move more slowly through the intestines, which is part of the reason that constipation is more common as one ages.

Dysphagia, abnormal swallowing, prevalence increases. Saliva levels diminish, resulting in a decreased ability to lubricate the food and an impaired ability to swallow. Loss of teeth and the use of dentures decrease the ability of the individual to chew food. Food that is not chewed well has a tendency to get stuck in the throat. The contraction ability of the esophagus, which connects the mouth to the stomach, weakens with age.

KIDNEY AND URINARY SYSTEM: The kidneys shrink. Starting at the age of thirty, the filtering process of the kidneys declines. Reductions in the number and functionality of nephrons, tiny tubes responsible for filtering the waste products from the body, are responsible.

Changes in the urinary system contribute to incontinence. The bladder holds less urine and has increased muscle contractions, which contributes to leaking. Females are prone to problems of the urinary system due to childbirth and decreased level of hormones. Childbirth causes trauma to the urinary tract that can lead to dysfunction as one ages. Decreased levels of sex hormones, which occur after menopause, adversely affect the urinary tract.

ENDOCRINE SYSTEM: The endocrine system produces chemical messengers called hormones to help the body regulate many of its processes. Glands dispersed throughout the body release hormones into the blood, where other organs use them. The endocrine system affects many body processes including sugar utilization, metabolism, growth, the thyroid, water balance, and electrolyte balance.

In aging, levels of hormones may increase, decrease, or stay the same. Disease states—such as diabetes, thyroid disease, high blood pressure, and osteoporosis—are affected by the endocrine system.

Immune System: Aging causes this system to be less effective, but most people have only subtle changes. Generally, the body is less able to fight infection. The body is also more prone to attack itself, resulting in a higher prevalence of disorders called autoimmune disease. The immune system is partly responsible for fighting cancer cells, resulting in an increased incidence of cancer as one ages. The ability to heal wounds also decreases.

Nervous System: The brain and spinal cord—two major sections of the nervous system—decrease in size; nerves also shrink in size and number.

Brain function slows as one ages, resulting in subtle changes such as difficulty with learning and forgetfulness. The brain loses nerve cells, but the effect this has on mental function is unclear.

Mental Health: The incidence of depression and dementia increases with aging. Attention, verbal smoothness, and logical analysis decline, while vocabulary can increase. Many functions of cognition remain stable, including communication skills, attention span, and visual perception. Many psychological conditions are more common in the older population, partly because they are brought out by declines in health. For example, as people with macular degeneration lose their eyesight, they will become more dependent on caregivers. This increased dependence is a common precursor of depression or anxiety.

Goals of Aging

The two major goals of healthy aging are:

- Delaying death
- Increasing the enjoyment you get out of life

Preventing disease and managing chronic disease prolongs life. The system outlined in the next chapter helps ensure that you are communicating effectively with your health care team and thereby managing chronic disease.

The ability to perform enjoyable activities defines good quality of life. A long life is not desirable if quality of life is poor. Poor control of chronic disease is one factor that leads to a reduced quality of life. The older population is a sick population; 80 percent of people over the age of sixty-five have at least one chronic disease; 50 percent have at least two chronic diseases. Health care responsibility increases quality of life by reducing the burden of chronic disease.

Most individuals would not want to live past one hundred if they were to be completely dependent on someone else to care for them. This would also lead to significant burden on the working population to care for such a large numbers of older patients. If older patients overrun the health care system, their living conditions and the care they receive will be poor.

The example presented in the opening of this chapter highlights how aged individuals can succumb to disease. John's main sins were that he lived an inactive lifestyle and had weight gain. This was enough to cause other systems to fail, resulting in the appearance of disease. If John continued his active lifestyle, it is likely that he would not have had the problems that developed.

Functional impairment may be the most important aspect of unhealthy aging. It is defined as a decline or inability in the capacity to perform tasks that are done routinely during the day such as bathing, dressing, using the toilet, preparing meals, taking medications as instructed, using the telephone, and maintaining finances. Functional impairment is increased as the number of chronic diseases increase. Arthritis, which affects over 50 percent of adults over the age of sixty-five, is a leading cause of functional impairment as it can lead to immobility, muscle wasting, and decreased ability to function on a day-to-day basis. All chronic disease process affects functional ability, with some resulting in more impairment than others.

Functional impairment is rarely related to one cause. The case in the beginning of the chapter is a story of how the aged body needs attention through health care responsibility, or functional impairment will ensue with the development of chronic diseases. Arthritis, deconditioning, stroke with left sided weakness, a broken hip, Parkinson's disease, depression, osteoporosis, and hypertension hamper the man. If only one disease state was present, he could compensate better, but multiple problems result in global impairment. This individual could also be said to have gone from a state of good health to becoming a frail person in a short period of time.

Frailty, a common term used in the medical community, is a loss in the ability to fight off stresses that lead to disability such as generalized weakness, immobility, frequent falls, weight loss, muscle wasting, poor exercise tolerance, incontinence, and frequent exacerbations of chronic disease. Frailty needs to be protected against through healthy lifestyles and disease management strategies.

Summary

The population is getting older and sicker. It is easy for individuals to get lost in the shuffle of the busy health care system. Older Americans are at increased risk for death and disability and need to assume responsibility for their personal well-being.

Each individual needs to understand the aging process and what he or she can do to minimize the effects of aging on the body. Without effort, the body is bound to age in a very unhealthy manner.

Healthy aging is defined as a postponement or decrease in the undesirable effects of aging and the ability to maintain optimal function. It involves maintaining physical and mental health, avoiding disease and maintaining independence. Getting quality health care is a key component to aging successfully.

The remainder of this book will teach you how to interact with the system to get the best care available. Practicing good preventative health care, communicating with the system, and partnering with your doctor to manage your health and diseases will reduce the impact aging has on quality and quantity of life.

SECTION 2

SURVIVING THE HEALTH CARE SYSTEM

CHAPTER 4

COMMUNICATION: YOUR KEY TO SUCCESS IN HEALTH CARE

Kristen is a sixty-five-year-old female with multiple medical problems including high blood pressure, heart disease, diabetes, arthritis, osteoporosis, glaucoma, cataracts, and an underactive thyroid gland. She would meet with her primary health care provider two times a year. Her doctor had multiple things that needed to be accomplished during their fifteen-minute visits. He needed to write prescriptions, fill out forms for her insurance company, and get notes from her heart doctor and diabetes specialist. The doctor was under tight time restrictions. Kristen was rarely organized and was unable to formulate responses to simple questions asked by her doctor. The doctor knew she was unable to present an accurate description of her medical problems and consequently chose his questions very carefully. This resulted in a limited exam and compromised her health care.

If Kristen was organized for her appointments and able to communicate effectively, her visits would be much smoother. Being able to relay a concise medical history, description of her current problems, updates from her cardiologist and diabetes doctor, and any medication changes would result in higher quality care. Knowing what tests she needs and when they were last taken would ensure that she would take advantage of all the medical technology available.

The effectiveness of any health care encounter is only as good as the interaction between the people involved. Each individual's health is a shared responsibility between the provider and the individual, but the only person you can control is yourself. Learning how to effectively communicate within the health care system can significantly enhance the quality of your health care.

Communicating with your doctor is an essential step in assuring good health. Doctors can make a diagnosis a majority of the time with a good description of the current problem without fancy medical tests. Because of this, most doctors say that taking a medical history is one of the most important parts of their job. Your ability to communicate with your doctor vastly improves your health care.

Delaying diagnosis is often the result of the patient not providing a good history. Prompt attention to any medical concerns is an important consideration in getting an accurate and timely diagnosis. Often, the diagnosis is missed because the patient does a poor job at describing the symptoms or not asking the right questions.

The Patient's Role

Multiple medical problems compounded with multiple medicines highlight the challenges of the doctors caring for older adults. It is critical for the older adult to provide an accurate history and course of his present illness.

Health care involves shared responsibility for decisions. Each consumer must comply with the mutually agreed upon plan of care. It is important that each individual is prepared for each encounter with the health care system and communicates in a concise way.

Components of Good Communication: Preparation and Organization

Proper communication requires preparation and organization. You would not go into a major speech without outlining what you were going to say; therefore, you should not go into a situation where your life is on the line such as a doctor's appointment without knowing what you are going to say.

The doctor will be able to do a better job if you are organized. While certain places such as emergency rooms are more difficult to prepare for, some basic principles apply to each health care encounter.

Three components are essential to preparing for a doctor's visit: personal medical record, visit form, and question form. The personal medical record (which is discussed at length in Chapter 11) is a concise way to prepare and report your history. The visit form is a specific form for the individual appointment. The form is in Appendix B and is explained in detail later in this chapter. The question form is used to record questions you have for your health care provider.

Preparing your personal health record is a cornerstone to getting good medical care. The personal health record (which will be detailed in Chapter 11) is a detailed account of your history. By preparing and organizing this information, you enhance your doctor's ability to care for you.

Preparing for a doctor's appointment with the use of the appropriate visit form assures your agenda is covered. Patients see the doctor under three broad circumstances: an acute illness, follow-up, and a routine maintenance exam. Learning how to organize information for each of these appointments improves your health care.

Doctors have limited time set aside for each appointment. Many individuals ramble on about multiple insignificant points, putting them at significant risk for receiving poor health care. Being organized helps ensure that you take advantage of the great health care that is available.

Making a diagnosis is difficult. Contrary to what most people think, medicine is not an exact science. It is possible for one patient to present five different doctors with same complaint and get five different answers.

Many patients have one or two symptoms and it is up to the doctor to determine the diagnosis and treatment. It is essential that each patient provide as much information as possible to make the diagnosis as easy as possible for the physician.

When talking about symptoms, be clear, objective, truthful, and persistent. Many health concerns are sensitive and embarrassing, but without all the details, the doctor will not be able to care for you properly. Do not let embarrassment be a barrier to communication with your doctor. If you do not want something to appear in the medical record, let the doctor know.

Be prepared to get all the necessary answers during your appointment. The visit forms listed in appendix B will guide you. Get instructions in writing from your doctor or use a tape recorder. If possible, bring a friend to write down the doctor's instructions for you. Understand your diagnosis and treatment so that you can participate in regaining your health. Patients need to be allies in their health care and to be given a clear account of the doctor's diagnosis and treatment. Understand what follow-up is needed.

The third component is preparing a list of questions prior to the appointment. List your most important concerns first as it is possible that you will not get to ask all of your questions. Make two copies of your question list so you can give one to your doctor.

You do not have to accept a particular diagnosis or treatment. If you do not agree with a specific treatment, ask the doctor for another solution or a consultation with another doctor. There is usually more than one way to handle any specific disease, and you have a right to know all of the alternatives. The doctor will view it negatively if you challenge everything he or she says, but this does not mean you cannot ask questions. Phrase questions constructively and with the purpose of enhancing your understanding of the condition or treatment.

Calling the Doctor

Preparation before calling the office results in better phone conversations. Write down a brief description of your concern and list two to three questions. If you have more than two to three questions or a complicated concern, you will be better served by making an office visit. Doctors receive many calls and will not personally handle every one; the office staff or one of the nurses can answer many questions. Receptionists and nurses collect the proper information and determine if a return call from the doctor is necessary. After talking to a receptionist or nurse, if you still believe it is necessary to speak with the doctor that is the time to ask.

Have a pen and paper available when calling the office. Emergency calls should be made as early in the day as possible so you can be scheduled in if necessary. Calls about less urgent matters could be delayed until midmorning.

When calling for a prescription refill, have the pharmacy phone number available. Make the request before you are out of pills so the doctor can review your record to see if the medication is still needed or if you need an office visit to reevaluate the need for the medication. If you call outside office hours, you risk getting a covering doctor.

Visiting Your Doctor: The Office Visit

To make a medical practice financially feasible, most office visits are only set up for ten to fifteen minutes. In that time, your provider needs to review the chart, take a patient history, examine you, explain his or her findings, and write a progress note and prescription if necessary.

To assure that your agenda is covered, it is essential that as a health care consumer you are prepared for the appointment. If you are not an active partner, you are guaranteed to get suboptimal care.

STEPS TO PREPARING AND ORGANIZING FOR YOUR VISIT

Helpful tips when visiting your health care provider

- Be on time. Being late to an appointment compromises the amount of time you have to spend with the health care provider and may result in a cancellation. The health care provider has a busy practice and being on time shows him or her that you value his or her time and your health.

- Get to know your doctor. Having a personal relationship with the provider can have a positive impact on the care that you receive.

- Give a good history. Prepare for the visit so you can provide the doctor with an accurate description of your problem or concerns. An accurate history is the most valuable tool a doctor has in making a diagnosis.

- Use the form in Appendix B or tape recorder to capture comments made by the doctor.

- Wear glasses and hearing aids to assure you see and hear everything the doctor demonstrates or says.

- Bring someone with you to be an extra set of eyes and ears.

- Talk openly about alcohol, tobacco, and lifestyle changes.

- Ask the health care provider to slow down or speak up if needed.

- Ask doctor to explain things in plain English.

- Bring in one page of organized questions in order of importance with a copy for your health care provider.

- Bring in your personal health care record.

- Ask the health care provider for copies of tests and lab work.

- Make sure that you understand what the doctor is saying to you. Repeat the important information back to him or her in your own words to assure you understand what was said.

QUESTION YOUR DOCTOR

Before leaving the office, make sure that you understand what the doctor thinks is causing your problem and what the treatment plan is. Table 4-1 suggests some questions to ask when you are presenting with a new problem or diagnosis.

Asking questions about medical testing and treatments helps assure you are a partner in your care. Testing is done so routinely in health care that it often is not questioned. Medical testing and treatments involve risk and it is important to discuss this in detail with your provider. More testing is not necessarily better; sometimes, waiting out symptoms may be a better option. When a new test is ordered ask the questions listed in Table 4-2.

It is important to have a full understanding about the treatments that the doctor orders. Table 4-3 provides a list of questions to ask when a new treatment is ordered. Medications are commonly prescribed to treat a specific diagnosis. Chapter 7 provides questions and suggestions for discussions when new medications are prescribed.

TABLE 4-1
WHEN PRESENTING WITH A NEW PROBLEM OR A NEW DIAGNOSIS

- What is causing my problem?

- Could more than one disease be causing my problem?

- How will this disease progress/What is my prognosis?

- What symptoms should I watch out for?

- What should I do for if these symptoms persist?

TABLE 4-2
WHEN NEW TESTS ARE ORDERED

- Is this the best test to evaluate my problem?

- What preparation should I make for the test?

- What is the possibility that this test will not affect treatment or diagnosis?

- How accurate are the tests?

- Is the test safe?

- What are the risks?

TABLE 4-3
WHEN NEW TREATMENT IS ORDERED

- What is the treatment?

- What is the chance the treatment will cure my disease or treat my signs and symptoms?

- What is the plan if this treatment does not work?

- What are the benefits and risks of the treatments?

- Can the treatment you are prescribing interact with any of the other medicines I am on?

- How should I take this medicine, with food/on an empty stomach?

- What are the side effects of this medicine?

DIFFERENT TYPES OF HEALTH CARE ENCOUNTERS

Step number two in preparing for your visit involves giving a concise history of your current concern. This section of the chapter provides a framework for you to organize and communicate your concerns under the three types of office visits: acute problems, follow-ups, and maintenance visits.

The most important part of an office visit is preparation. Use the steps below to optimize your appointment time.

- Bring your personal medical record to each appointment.

- Accurately describe signs and symptoms. Use the form in Appendix B that best describes the type of office visit you are having.

- Prepare a list of questions (Use question form in Appendix B) in order of importance with a copy for you and your doctor.

- Keep it short and sweet. Stay focused on your problem.

COMMUNICATING WITH YOUR HEALTH CARE PROVIDERS

ACUTE VISITS

Acute visits involve specific complaints. Common examples of acute visits are cold symptoms, fever, stomach pain, diarrhea, constipation, and weight loss. Use this visit to focus on the current problem; don't discuss other problems. Acute visits are usually short, often only ten minutes. Use that time wisely. Table 4-4 provides steps in preparing for an acute visit.

Come to the appointment prepared. Filling out the acute visit form (in Appendix B) before the appointment assures proper information is transmitted to your provider. If you are acutely ill, a prepared history can significantly enhance the doctor's ability to accurately diagnosis and treat the problem.

The next part of the acute visit is the physical exam. If the history and physical are inconclusive, diagnostic tests are ordered. Many of these tests can be eliminated with the use of a good history and physical exam. No test is without risk including immediate risk from the test such as risk of infection with a simple blood draw or long-term risk such as exposure to radiation from X-rays and CAT scans. Question your health care provider about the need for any diagnostic test using the questions listed in Table 4-3.

TABLE 4-4
STEPS IN PREPARING FOR AN ACUTE VISIT

1. In advance, complete the acute visit form from Appendix B.

2. Record the date and the doctor's name.

3. Describe why you are seeing the doctor.

4. Describe your symptoms. Complete the information form in appendix B for the complaint you are presenting with.

5. While at the appointment, record the doctor's diagnosis on the form.

6. Record the treatment, including medications ordered, how to take the medications, and side effects.

7. Record any follow-up recommended by the doctor including when to follow up, any situations that would require you to follow up sooner, and any information the doctor wants you to track to aid in the evaluation of the effectiveness of treatment.

8. Record any testing recommended by the doctor.

FOLLOW-UP VISITS

Follow-up visits are appointments that take place to check on an acute or chronic problem. It is important to have an understanding of the type of information the doctor needs from you to make a full assessment of the problem. For example, for someone with diabetes, the doctor will want to see blood sugar results that the patient has obtained with the use of a monitor.

How do patients know what information is needed? They ask. Every time that you have an appointment with your provider, ask what type of follow-up is required. Record on the acute visit form when your follow-up appointment is and what type of follow-up information that the doctor requests for that visit.

Every chronic condition should prompt a question to your doctor about the type of follow-up you require. Examples of follow-up information you can get for your doctor include blood pressure readings if you are afflicted with high blood pressure or daily weigh-ins if you have the diagnosis of congestive heart failure.

MAINTENANCE VISITS

Maintenance visits do not focus on any one problem or disease state but look at your overall health. They are key components to good health. These visits assure that preventative health care screenings, lifestyle, medications, and overall health are optimized. Based on the findings of this exam, more intensive testing or examinations may take place in the form of a follow-up visit. The most common maintenance visit is the annual exam. Another maintenance exam is the initial visit with a new health care provider.

ANNUAL VISIT

Annual visits assure optimal health. The annual visit entails a history and physical exam and review of medications. It ensures your entire preventative health care measures are up to date. Schedule this appointment at a time when you are not sick so that this appointment focuses on your overall health picture and not on an acute illness. Doctors are unable to handle too many health problems at one visit.

Older individuals are at increased risk for many chronic diseases and it is important that they are monitored for regularly. Health care providers are often very busy and do not take the time to adequately test you for diseases that are in the early stages. The disease states only get worse if they go undetected. Helping the health care provider with disease detection – by following guidelines for preventative health care screenings - is the only way to assure you are properly monitored.

The annual form in Appendix B will guide you through the steps to assure your total health picture is evaluated. Before the appointment, complete the annual visit form, including recording any symptoms that you are having and their descriptions; social questions; the depression screen; and the functional assessment. Lastly, assure that the steps at the bottom of page three of the annual visit form are completed during the visit. Do not rely solely on your doctor—help your doctor care for you appropriately.

INITIAL VISIT

The first visit with a new health care provider is a time when a patient needs to convey a complete medical history. The completeness of this history is essential to receive quality care. Health care providers need a plethora of information about you including: past diseases, surgeries, family history, social history, medications, medication allergies, and many other items to provide safe care. The individual who has lived over fifty years often has a complex medical history. Without preparation before the appointment, it is not possible to convey accurate information to the new health care provider.

Maintaining a personal health care record (which will be described in Chapter 11) significantly aids this process. It allows you to record all vital medical information. Bringing a copy of this information assists your health care provider in giving you the best care possible. Bring a completed copy of the annual evaluation form to the initial visit. A health care provider on an annual basis, including at the initial evaluation, should evaluate all items on the annual visit form.

SPECIAL SITUATIONS

EMERGENCY ROOM

It is more difficult to prepare for a visit to the emergency room or an urgent care clinic. Patients being treated in these situations are usually acutely ill and are in no condition to prepare an extensive list of questions and describe symptoms in detail.

Going to the emergency room accompanied by a loved one or friend significantly improves your care. This individual helps you transmit information to the emergency room staff. If you are unable to bring your personal health care record, this individual can bring it along for you. While waiting for the doctor and nurses, take some time to fill out one of the acute care visit forms. This gives you an opportunity to think about your current problem and transmit proper information.

Emergency room personnel are likely unfamiliar with your past medical history. While in the emergency room, you are often too sick to remember exact details of your medical history. The personal medical record guarantees your history is transmitted accurately.

The emergency room form, in Appendix B, allows you to capture information obtained in the emergency room for your personal health care record. It will help your primary care doctor understand what happened in the emergency room. Patients typically have follow-up visits with their primary doctor after an ER visit. Poor communication between the emergency room and the primary doctor is the norm. By gathering all the necessary information, you can greatly enhance this communication process and improve your care.

If possible when going to the emergency room, bring:

- Your personal medical record

- A loved one or friend

- The ER form in Appendix B

- The acute visit form in Appendix B. You can fill this out while you are waiting to be seen.

SPECIALIST

Specialty visits are initiated when the primary care doctor can't handle a problem. The specialist needs a comprehensive medical history, so bring your personal health care record.

This also may be an acute visit if a new problem is being evaluated or a follow-up visit if the specialist is following up on a problem the primary doctor is evaluating. When you are going to visit the specialist for the first time:

1. Bring your personal health care record.

2. Ask the doctor who referred you about the information the specialist will need. For example, if a cardiologist is seeing you, the doctor will need an accurate description of your symptoms, blood pressure read-

ings, any labs you have had, and any diagnostic tests already performed such as a stress test.

3. Ask your doctor to fill out a referral form listed in Appendix B to aid the specialist in caring for you.

4. Gather any information for the specialist appointment. For example, if you are seeing a lung doctor for cough, stomach doctor for abdominal pain or a heart doctor for chest pain, use the acute care form and acute care describing information in Appendix B.

5. If being seen for follow-up on a chronic problem, provide the doctor with any information you can. If a heart doctor for high blood pressure is seeing you, provide a record of blood pressures; if a diabetes specialist is seeing you, provide a list of your blood sugars. For more complete information on chronic disease tracking forms, visit http://www.hcrbooks.com.

6. Bring a self-addressed stamped envelope for the doctor to send you a copy of his or her progress note and any test results. Give this to the doctor or his nurse at the end of the appointment. Remind the receptionist on the way out that you want information sent to you. Add his or her note in your personal medical record. Your primary doctor will be very impressed when you present him or her with a copy of the specialist's progress note. It will also make the doctor's job easier.

Health Care Responsibility: Communicate Efficiently By

1. Having a firm grasp on your medical history by completing the personal health care record (*see Chapter 11*).

2. Organizing a concise history of your concern by preparing the forms outlined at the end of this chapter for each health care encounter.

3. Understanding the chronic diseases that you have. Learning about transmission of specific health care information related to common chronic disease can be enhanced by visiting http://www.hcrbooks.com.

4. Knowing what questions to ask your health care provider. This chapter provides some general questions. Lists of questions throughout the book will guide you in communicating with your health care provider.

CHAPTER 5

HOSPITALIZATION

The Institute of Medicine estimates that in 1999, 44,000 to 98,000 Americans die each year due to mistakes in the hospital.[1] In addition to death, other complications and increased health care costs contribute to the dire state of the American hospital system. Complications, including errors, cost the system billions of dollars each year.

Hospitalization is often necessary when individuals are acutely ill, but it is fraught with risks. This chapter discusses the risks and ways to avoid complications and errors. Each individual needs to be organized during his or her hospital stay and be involved in the care.

The hospital is an environment in which people, especially older people, lose their sense of identity. Patients are thrown out of their daily routine, not eating their own food, not sleeping in their own beds, and not taking their own medicine.

RISKS OF THE HOSPITAL

The hospital is a dangerous place. The risks of hospitalization can be subdivided into complications, errors, and iatrogenic disease (disease produced by doctors or other health care workers).

You may be thinking, "Doctors don't cause disease." Yes, they do. They rarely do this purposely but doctors and health care providers frequently cause disease unintentionally. Examples include infections, side effects or complications of medication, and major bleeding or kidney failure from a diagnostic procedure.

COMPLICATIONS

Complications, or negative events that occur during the hospital stay, are more common in the older population. Risk factors for complications to occur include: being a nursing home resident, increased number of medications, poor health, longer hospital stays, greater than age 75, dementia, inability to perform activities of daily living such as bathing or grooming, and poor physical functioning such the inability to walk independently.

Common complications include: sun downing, falls, excessive bed rest, pressure sores, malnutrition, and increased dependency. Sun downing, which commonly occurs in those with dementia, is an increased amount of confusion often associated with agitation or other behavior disturbances that occur at nighttime. Those without diagnosed dementia who suffer sun downing in a new environment are often diagnosed shortly thereafter with dementia. Sun downing can result in falls, use of restraints (tying the patient down), or excessive use of medicine to control behaviors.

Sometimes bed rest is necessary, but usually getting patients up and moving is the best strategy to prevent complications. Bed rest breeds dependency, which leads to further complications including debility. The risk is even greater in those who are older and have a baseline lower level of functioning.

Pressure sores, more commonly known as bedsores, are a frequent complication of prolonged hospitalization due to bed rest, poor nutrition, and dehydration. Pressure sores can be prevented with good nursing care. If you have not been getting up while hospitalized, ask the nursing staff if you can get out of bed. If you are unable to get out of bed, make sure you are getting turned frequently (at least every two hours) or placed on a specialty mattress to reduce pressure on areas of your body.

Hospitalized patients are sick, and may not be eating well. In addition, disease states increase the rate at which your body uses energy, so eating the amount of food you normally eat may not be enough to maintain body weight and promote healing. Bringing your own food can sometimes prevent not only malnutrition but also other illness and expense. Before doing this, always check with your provider, as many hospitalized individuals require special diets. For example, after a stroke patients often need food that is puréed to prevent the food from sliding down into the lungs and causing pneumonia.

Falls are a frequent occurrence among hospitalized patients due to weakness from illness, mobility restriction from intravenous lines, sedation due to new medicines, and getting up to go to the bathroom without assistance. Often, falls result from a combination of factors such as weakness secondary to the disease for which the patient was admitted and lack of familiarity with the environment. New medications can lead to falls. For example, new blood pressure pills can result in dizziness or unsteadiness. Water pills can lead to increased urination, especially at night. When the urge to urinate comes on at night, a patient trying to maneuver to the bathroom in an unfamiliar environment increases risk of falls.

Taking responsibility for your safety consists of asking for help when ambulating and knowing the medicines you are on and the risk they pose for falls.

MEDICATION ERRORS

Complications from medicine can be broken down into errors and side effects. Many times, side effects are expected but the doctor decides that the risk is worth the benefit of the treatment. All medicines have side effects, but some are much more dangerous than others. When taking new medicines, report unusual sensations to your doctor or nurse. For example:

- Antibiotic can cause an infection of the intestines resulting in diarrhea or yeast infections.

- Powerful antibiotics such as gentamicin or tobramycin can cause kidney damage or hearing loss.

- Heart medicines are a very broad class but any new drug for the heart needs to be monitored closely for side effects including low blood pressure, falls, or dehydration.

- Some pain medicines—called nonsteroidal anti-inflammatory medicine—can cause stomach bleeding or kidney shutdown.

- Other pain medicines such as narcotics can cause confusion, dizziness, and falls.

- Prednisone, a steroid, is used to treat inflammation such as certain types of arthritis or lung diseases and can thin bones, raise blood sugar, or cause weight gain.

- Cancer drugs have many side effects and can damage many body systems.

Errors

Medication errors are not unusual in the hospital. Patients are often admitted by a physician who is unfamiliar with his or her medical history. Therefore, the admitting doctor relies solely on the patient's report of medications when prescribing medications. If the patient does not provide an accurate list of medications, then he or she may not get all of the medications necessary.

Accurately reporting the medications that a hospitalized patient is currently taking is a critical step in preventing errors. This is best accomplished by providing the admitting doctor with your personal health care record.

Patients who get the wrong medications are another form of error common in hospitalized patients. Nurses are very busy and care for multiple patients with whom they are unfamiliar. The best way to prevent this is to keep track of the medicines you take. Maintaining the hospital chart, which is listed in Appendix B and described in detail later, is one method to track your medications.

Misdiagnosis

Medicine is not an exact science; it is a combination of art and science. Coming up with the correct diagnosis is important to prevent progression of disease and the possible death and disability that can accompany disease. Some diseases are more easily diagnosed than others. Cooperation from the patient can significantly aid the doctor in making a speedy and accurate diagnosis. Accurately reporting of the medical history and current symptoms, asking the right questions, and making sure you are getting optimal care reduce the chance your doctor will diagnose you incorrectly.

DISCHARGE

Upon discharge from the hospital, patients receive instructions including a list of medications. Comparing this list of medicine to the personal hospital chart that you have been keeping during your stay can aid you in assuring there are no errors. If the lists do not match up, ask the discharge nurse or the doctor for clarification. Patients may assume that medications not on the list were discontinued in the hospital. Many times this is the case, but many times medications were accidentally left off. Oversights and omissions occur even with the best-intentioned health care providers. Your best defense is to closely monitor your medical care. No one has your best interest in mind more than you.

Discharge instructions should include a scheduled appointment with your doctor or a number to call to set up that appointment. Make sure that this appointment is carried out. This can mean the difference between life and death. New medications are often started in the hospital and require outpatient monitoring to assure they are not only effective but also are not causing any life-threatening complications.

DISCHARGE STEPS

1. Ask every day when discharge will occur. The answer to this question may not be known, but it is important that you are prepared for discharge.

2. Meet with the doctor before you are discharged. Make sure a family member or loved one is with you to be an extra set of ears.

3. Ask the doctor to review the medication list and compare this with your hospitalized list of medication. If there is any discrepancy, question the doctor.

4. Ask the doctor to confirm follow-up appointments, when they are needed and with whom.

5. Ask the doctor what symptoms would require medical attention and what to do if they occur.

6. Ask what your recovery will entail.

7. Ask how the doctor may be reached.

Iatrogenic Disease Infections

Two million hospitalized patients suffer from hospital-acquired infections each year.[2] Hospital-induced infections are also known as nosocomial infections. They not only increase the cost and length of your stay but also increase the risk of dying in the hospital. Nosocomial infections cost the health care system billions of dollars a year. Infection rates vary by hospital, so it is important to be informed about which hospitals are riskiest. Contact your local health department to determine which hospitals have the lowest incidences of these infections.

The most common types of hospital-acquired infections are urinary tract infections, severe diarrhea, pneumonia, and blood infections. Hospitals have bacteria and viruses that most patients have not been exposed to previously. And, most hospitalized patients have a suppressed immune system due to their illness and have a more difficult time fighting infections. Many of these infections can be prevented. The most important step is to make sure everyone who gets close to you washes his or her hands.

Invasive procedures—actions where some type of instrument is introduced into the body—may initiate infection. Examples procedures include urinary catheterization, intravenous lines insertions, and cardiac catheterizations. These procedures are done by busy nurses and doctors who at times may not follow the proper techniques and may introduce bacteria into the body.

Infections often are spread from another sick patient. If your roommate is showing signs of an infectious disease, ask to move rooms. Signs include: coughing, diarrhea, runny nose, fever, or increased confusion. Many diseases are passed through the air or from touching something that the sick patient has touched, and being in close proximity to someone with infection increases the risk of disease.

Diagnostic Testing

Diagnostic tests have risks, including pain or discomfort, allergic reaction, bleeding or infection. It is imperative that you inquire about the necessity of each test that you have. A CAT scan can save your life but it also provides a tremendous amount of radiation, which is a potential deadly side effect.

X-rays sometimes are performed to help diagnosis or rule out pneumonia but they are often not needed. Someone who has a runny nose, sore throat, cough, and a low-grade fever for twenty-four hours and who on physical exam has completely normal lung sounds is very unlikely to have pneumonia. X-rays are generally safe tests, but they are not completely benign as they do entail radiation exposure.

A number of steps should be taken when diagnostic tests are recommended in the hospital. When the technician arrives, ask for whom the test is scheduled. Sometimes, tests are performed on the wrong people. When the test is recommended by your doctor, ask the questions listed in Table 5-1.

Table 5-1
Questions to Ask When a Diagnostic Test Is Ordered

- What is the purpose of this test?

- Is there any other way to gain this information?

- What is the probability this test will yield a diagnosis for my condition?

- Could we get by without the test?

- What is the preparation for this test?

- Is the test painful/uncomfortable?

- Who conducts the test?

- How is the test done?

- How long will it take to get results?

- How much experience do you have with this test?

- How expensive is this test? Will insurance pay for it?

- Are there any side effects?

- Will I be exposed to any radiation?

- What will happen if I do not have it done? (If you feel that the test is not in your best interest, you can refuse the test.)

- What is the false-positive and false-negative rate? (False positive is a situation when an individual has a positive finding but there is no disease present. Positive findings often require more tests, which are usually more invasive and carry more risks, to confirm or rule out the suspected disease.)

PREVENTING PROBLEMS IN THE HOSPITAL: YOUR ROLE

Some errors are just mistakes that you cannot do anything about, no matter how knowledgeable, attentive, or careful you are. On the other hand, many errors can be overcome by being an informed consumer, asking questions, and trusting your instincts. It is important that you take responsibility while you are in the hospital to reduce the risk of the above complications. An educated and prepared patient is the best protection against medical error.

The first step in preventing medical errors in the hospital is to ask your doctor about the possibility of being treated at home. Many times hospitalization is necessary, but there are times when being treated as an outpatient is possible. Avoiding the hospital eliminates the possibility of complications, errors, and adverse events.

FAMILY SUPPORT/PATIENT ADVOCATE

Family support is an important part of getting through the hospital experience with the best possible outcome. Family and friends can be advocates for you. They can be an extra set of ears, help you ask questions, and help provide reassurance.

Families and friends can be seen as an extra burden by the hospital staff, but this does not have to be the case. They need to be courteous and respectful. Hospitalizations are stressful times, and families can become frantic and abuse staffers who are just trying to do their jobs. Remaining calm and treating the staff with respect will go a lot further in assuring that you or your loved one gets good care than being rude and abrasive will. Bringing snacks into busy nurses and staff goes a long way. Providing a little bit of appreciation for the staff can help assure that your loved one gets some extra attention while in the hospital.

HOSPITAL CHART

To prevent errors and help the health care team, keep your own personal chart. Hospitalized patients are often not well enough to keep great notes on their illness, so it's helpful to involve a family member in this process.

Your hospital chart is nothing more than a couple pieces of paper where key information is recorded. The personal hospital chart includes seven sections to monitor and follow your hospital course. The form is found in Appendix B. Keep a copy by your bedside.

In the first section, record your doctors' names, how to contact them, and the times they make rounds. Every time you see a new doctor, record this information. It will allow you to keep information on not only your primary care doctor but also the specialists caring for you. Record information on the head nurse of the unit. Knowing who is in charge and how to contact him or her will help if a problem arises.

The second section is a place to record information about each doctor's visit. Each time you see a doctor, record the date and time in column number one and the name of the doctor in column two. The third column is for you to record any tests ordered and any comments that the doctor made. Feel free to use more than one row to record comments or information on testing.

The third section is where your list of medicines are recorded. Medications are common sources of errors in the hospital. Helping the nursing staff by keeping a record of what medicines you take and when you take them assures you will get the proper medicine. Keep in mind that there is some flexibility in the times nurses administer medicines. Nurses take care of multiple patients and are unable to give all 9:00 a.m. medicines to all of their patients at exactly 9 o'clock. One of the most common errors in the hospital is a missing medication dose. Patient vigilance decreases this risk. Ask the nurse for a copy of your medication list. Record it in section three of the chart. This list should match up with your list of home medicines but may include additions or deletions. Any medication that is on your hospital medication list but not on your home medication list or vice versa should be questioned. It may be a purposeful omission or addition, but it may not be.

On page two of the chart, record your medications, the dosages, and the times they are administered. You also need to know why they are administered. Understand why you are on the drugs, the side effects, and the length of treatment.

A drug sometimes omitted on hospital admission is antidepressants. After a few days being off this medicine, the patient can develop nausea, dizziness, and headache. However, providers may interpret these as new symptoms that need to be worked up and this can add to the number of days and dollars of your hospital visit. If you are not diligent about the medications you receive in the hospital, you could be looking at an extended stay.

In the fourth section, take notes on any new diagnoses. Basic information is recorded in section two, but this section allows more room for details. Always ask for any literature about these diseases, but do not neglect to take notes as your doctor will be able to tell you how this disease affects you. Studies indicate that patients forget most of what they are told immediately after it is told especially in a stressful situation such as the hospital.

In the fifth section, record more detailed information on blood work. Always ask doctor to give you information about your blood work. For example, ask, "What blood work did you perform today and what specifically did it show?" Ask for hard copies of laboratory tests. Later, these copies can be placed in your personal medical record.

In the sixth section, record information on testing performed during your hospitalization including X-rays, CAT scans, MRIs, ultrasounds, or cardiac procedures. Again, ask the doctor for specific information with questions such as "What did the CAT scan show?" Ask for a hard copy for your personal medical record.

In the seventh section, record information on any surgical procedures or other medical procedures. This could include a cardiac catheterization, thoracentesis, or biopsies. Ask the doctor for an interpretation and get a hard copy for your personal medical record.

In the next section, record a list of questions as they arise. Continually update the list of questions as patients never remember all of the questions that they want to ask the doctor. The section includes questions you should ask your doctor every day.

The last section is a general section where you can record general notes that do not fit anywhere else.

KEY POINTS

Below is a listing of the important steps to improve your health care while in the hospital.

- Avoid hospital care if at all possible.

- Bring your personal medical record, which includes your medication list.

- Keep your own medical chart. The form is provided in Appendix B or can be downloaded from http://www.hcrbooks.com.

- Insist that the doctors, nurses, aides, laboratory workers, and anyone who cares for you wash their hands. Put the sign up listed in Appendix B above your bed.

- When getting a pill, ask for the name and mark it off on your medical record.

- Be nice to the nursing staff.

- Assign a patient advocate, typically a family member or close friend, and have frequent visitors.

- If having surgery, make sure the proper area is marked. Talk to the surgeon and anesthesiologist.

- If there is a problem, voice it assertively but be kind. Show appreciation if it is remedied properly.

- Know your rights.

- Get a private room if possible, if insurance will cover the cost.

- At discharge, get your list of discharge medicines and compare them to you hospital chart. Discuss any discrepancies with staff before leaving the hospital.

CHAPTER 6

THE NURSING HOME

America is an aging society, and older individuals are at increased risk for nursing home placement partly because the incidence of chronic disease increases with age. Chronic diseases afflict many nursing home patients and often lead to disability and impair the ability to safely and effectively live independently.

WHEN DOES ONE NEED NURSING HOME PLACEMENT?

There are three classifications of nursing home patients: short-term stay patients, respite stay patients, and long-term care patients.

Short-term stay patients are broken down into rehabilitation stay patients and those who require intensive nursing care. Older individuals who fall at home and break a hip are likely to need therapy to regain their strength to live independently again. Rehabilitation stays in the nursing home have a goal of maximizing function. In addition to the hip fractures, there are many other types of patients who need rehabilitative nursing home stays such as those who have had a joint replacement or open-heart surgery or who have had a major medical illness with a prolonged hospital stay such as a stroke, heart attack, or prolonged bout of pneumonia. These patients also are usually afflicted with multiple chronic medical problems or an overall poor level of functioning.

Some individuals are in need of intensive nursing care for a specific medical concern. An infected wound in need of frequent dressing changes and intravenous antibiotics is a common reason for this type of nursing home stay. A doctor also can directly admit a patient from home if the doctor feels that treatment at home will be ineffective or unsafe but not serious enough to require hospitalization.

Respite stays are a short-term stays for patients. When caregivers need a break, they place residents in nursing facilities for a short period of time. The typical scenario involves demented patients being cared for at home. The family members go on a vacation and need a place for their loved one to stay. Since the patients are unable to live independently, they are placed in a nursing facility until the family members return from vacation.

Some individuals are unable to be cared for at home and need long-term placement in a nursing home. Long-term placement is needed when catastrophic medical issues occur or multiple chronic medical conditions add up. This can include someone who has had a catastrophic stroke and is in need of twenty-four-hour nursing care. It could include the patient with dementia and frequent wandering who is unsafe at home.

Here are some signs that a person living in the community needs long-term care:

- Taking medicine incorrectly such as taking too many or missing doses.

- Inattention to activities of daily living such as grooming, eating, decreased hygiene, or an unclean house.

- Changes in spending habits or not paying bills.

- Increased confusion such as forgetting how to use items, decreased ability to communicate, repeating questions, and getting lost.

- Strange behaviors such as wandering down the street in pajamas.

- Decreased cleanliness of the home.

- Smell of urine and feces in the home.

What to Look for in a Nursing Home

Below is a number of steps one should make to assure the proper nursing home is selected:

Preparation

1. List all the nursing homes that are convenient to your home.

2. Talk with nursing home staff, people who have had family members in nursing homes, doctors, the long-term care ombudsman, social workers, and clergy.

3. Review the nursing home site at www.medicare.gov/NHcompare/home.asp.

4. Narrow the list down to a few nursing homes to visit.

5. Visit the nursing homes on your list and observe/do the following:

   • Do patients look happy?

   • Is the building clean and well maintained?

   • Do patients just sit around and look bored?

   • Does the food look good?

   • Are call lights responded to quickly?

   • Does the staff looked stressed out?

   • Are staff members responsive to family and patient's needs and requests?

   • Are patients calling out for help?

   • Is there excessive noise?

   • Do patients smell clean? Are there any strong odors?

   • Ask to eat a meal.

Meet with the staff and ask:

- Do they have special services such as transportation services, a store, and beauty shop?

- What do you like about this place?

- What do you dislike about this place?

- Do you ever work short staffed?

- Do you like to eat here?

- Are snacks available for patients?

Ask family members of other patients or patients who are able to communicate:

- What do you like/dislike about this place?

- Are you glad you chose this place?

- Is staff helpful and caring?

- Are you invited to plan-of-care meetings?

- What happens when you have a problem?

- Is the food good and do you get enough?

- Does each shift have enough help?

- How often do they check on you?

W<small>HAT TO</small> E<small>XPECT IN THE</small> N<small>URSING</small> H<small>OME</small>

Nursing homes should provide a homelike environment where all of the activities of daily living are meet such as eating, bathing, and grooming.

Here is a list of things that should happen in a nursing home

- Safety/good medical care.

- Interaction with staff.

- Stimulation such as activities and games.

- Pleasant and safe environment

- Cleanliness and an odor-free environment

- Twenty-four-hour nursing care by nurses and nurses aides

- Therapy services such as physical therapy, occupation therapy, and speech therapy

- Evaluation of nutritional needs by a registered dietitian

- Access to social workers

- A doctor who is assigned as your primary doctor while you are at the nursing home. The doctor will see the patient around the admission time and then about one time a month. If there are medical problems that arise, the doctor is called and handles issues over the phone. No doctor is on site at all times. It is different than a hospital, where a doctor sees the patient every day.

The home is a "nursing" home. It is run mainly by nurses who provide nursing care and use nursing judgment to care for the patients.

TYPES OF NURSING HOME PATIENTS

SKILLED PATIENTS

Skilled patients are nursing home residents who have special needs and receive services that are paid for by insurance. Usually, these services are some form of therapy or intensive nursing care such as wound management or intravenous therapy. When you are maxed out on your therapy or no longer require intensive skilled nursing care, your skilled time will be over and insurance will not pay.

At this point, patients and their families have to decide where to go next. Many people will go home with some nursing care and therapy; others will go to an assisted living facility, where they still get some nursing care but are more independent. Some people need to stay in the nursing home on a long-term basis.

LONG-TERM PLACEMENT

Some individuals are not able to live in the community by themselves or have a significant disability that does not allow them to live with minimal care in an assisted living facility. They are debilitated to a point where the only safe way to live is with twenty-four-hour nursing support. The nursing home becomes the new home.

THE NURSING HOME EXPERIENCE

The nursing home can be a scary place, and having an understanding of what happens during a stay reduces trepidation. Nursing homes are not as comfortable as home, but they do not have to be unpleasant.

Admission to a nursing home is stressful and confusing. This is going to be the resident's new home over the next few weeks to months or maybe even permanently. Having some knowledge about the nursing home procedure can cut down on some of the anxiety.

Here are some things to know when you are admitted to a nursing home.

- Orders are sent by your doctor to the nursing home.

- These orders are reviewed by the nursing staff who do a complete nursing assessment.

- The nursing staff adds orders, after the patient is evaluated.

- These orders are then approved by the doctor.

- Your doctor at the nursing home may not be your primary care doctor.

- Your nursing home doctor will visit soon after admission, and then every thirty to sixty days. Nursing homes can handle many medical conditions including common urinary tract infections, pneumonias, dehydration, and minor traumas. If you are sick enough to be seen by a doctor, you are sent to the emergency room.

- Most patients are evaluated by physical therapy, occupational therapy, and speech therapy specialists. If the patients qualify, they will be picked up by the different therapy services.

- Your diet will be evaluated by a dietitian. Three meals a day and snacks will be provided.

- You will be cared for on a day-to-day basis by a team of nurses and nurses aides.

- You will not be provided with one-on-one care. The nurse and nurses aide who are assigned to you will care for many other patients.

- A nursing support team will evaluate all of your needs to help assure that you are getting optimal care.

- Social workers are available to assure your social needs are cared for such as discharge planning.

- If you have to go out to doctor appointments, the nursing home can arrange transportation through a local ambulance company.

- Most nursing homes have a variety of doctors who can see you, including psychiatrists, psychologists, podiatrists, dentists, eye doctors, and sometimes ear/nose/throat doctors.

- Many nursing homes hire nurse practitioners or physician assistants who are on site forty hours a week. These advanced practitioners have higher-level skills and are able to diagnosis and treat common medical problems.

What Happens after You Settle In?

The nursing home has multiple team members to help the patient meet his or her goals. The director of nursing will oversee all aspects of nursing care. Bigger nursing homes also have assistant directors of nursing. One nurse oversees each unit. Staff nurses supervise the multiple nursing aides who are assigned to each unit and are responsible for most of the day-to-day care such as bathing, hygiene, and feeding.

In addition to the direct care nurses, there are review nurses who spend their days making sure the patients are hitting their goals. These review nurses examine patients, review records, and talk with families, nurses, and therapists to help assure patients receive optimal care. These nurses help assure that patients receive appropriate exercise, nutrition, laboratory follow-up, and medications.

Administrators oversee the facility. They are responsible for managing the finances, setting and enforcing policy, and supervising personnel. Large nursing homes have an assistant administrator.

The dietary staff is responsible for getting food to the patient. The dietitian is responsible for assuring all patients get the proper diet. The dietary manager oversees the kitchen. Cooks are in charge of preparing the food while nurses aides and nurses are accountable for assuring that patients get their food.

Social workers help with discharge to make sure all the services are set up for home, including therapies, nursing care, and any other services that are needed. Social workers are responsible for setting up family meetings with long-term residents and coordinating services.

The activities department sets up games, organizes spiritual activities, plans day trips, and keeps patients active and happy.

Therapists help get patients back on their feet. Physical therapists restore physical function and help with locomotion. Occupational therapists help individuals regain their ability to perform activities of daily living such as eating, grooming, and dressing. Speech therapist help individuals with swallowing and cognitive function.

The attending physician is one of the least involved members of the team, but is responsible for the overall care of the patient. Attending physicians are not on site all the time; many only come into the facility when they have new admissions or perform their regulatory visits, which need to occur every thirty to sixty days.

Each patient has a periodic care conferences to discuss his or her strengths, weakness, diagnoses, goals, and treatments. Families and patients are invited to attend these meetings. The first of these conferences is scheduled shortly after admission and then at least every three months thereafter.

Discharge planning is done at a meeting with the nursing home team. At these meetings it is decided whether the patient has met his or her goals and could function safely at home. Where the patient would be discharged is also discussed. Common places include home, home with another family member, assisted living, or long-term residency in the nursing home. Sometimes, prior to discharge the occupational therapist does a home evaluation to assure that the residence is set up safely for the patient. Social workers set up home health nursing, therapy services if needed, and medications. Follow-up with the primary care medical provider is another task that is scheduled upon discharge from the nursing home.

How to Make the Most of Your Nursing Home Stay and Practice Health Care Responsibility

Nursing homes are not like home, and patient expectations are often not in line with reality. Patients and or families come in for their preadmission tour, which is essential a sales pitch, and nursing homes put their best foot forward and make things look better than they are.

Many patients and families expect many things to be the same as the hospital when entering the nursing home. While patients are sick in the nursing home, they are not as acutely ill as they are in the hospital. Hospitals are staffed much more intensively than nursing homes and, consequently, care is different. Hospitals are reimbursed much better than nursing homes. Each nursing home nurse is assigned to approximately twenty patients while each hospital nurse is assigned one to five patients. The ratio of nursing aides to patients is lower in the hospital.

When a call light goes off in the hospital, the response time is very rapid but in the nursing home it takes much longer. However, nursing homes are usually more "homey" than hospitals.

Nursing home placement is a stressful time. Patients and family members want their loved ones to get better, and this is often a slow process. Frustration is common because progress is not made quickly. Nursing home patients are usually older with multiple medical problems and do not have the physical reserve to bounce back from an illness that people in their twenties do. Nursing homes are not staffed to care for patients as an attentive family member could at home. When nursing home residents ring the call light, there is usually a delay before a staffer comes to their rooms.

If nursing homes do not provide attentive care, why go? Nursing homes offer the advantage of twenty-four-hour care with specialty equipment and specialty staff that is not available at home.

Here is a list of things that patients and families can do to make the most of a nursing home experience.

- Have a power of attorney. This allows someone to make legal decisions if you are not competent to make decisions. It also helps to decrease or avoid family conflicts. The social worker in the nursing home can point you in the right direction to getting a power of attorney set up. It usually requires that you go through an attorney's office.

- Learn about your medical conditions and treatments and progression of the disease. Nursing home patient are typically chronically ill, and it is essential that you have a complete understanding of your health and overall prognosis. Nursing home staff, especially an advanced practice nurse or the doctor, can help you with this.

- Know your health care provider's schedule. Talk with him or her about your overall health.

- Be nice to the nursing staff. Staff has to care for a number of patients; they will not care for you or like you would get cared for by an attentive family member. If there is a problem, voice it right away. But don't be hypercritical; no one wants to deal with a finicky family or patient. Compliment the staff at every opportunity. Have family bring in snacks for the nursing home staff, such as cookies or candy. This can go along way in getting great care.

- Learn Medicare/Medicaid rules; know the appeals process and how to challenge the nursing home decisions regarding limitations to therapies and skilled time, which are paid by insurance.

- Give yourself time to adjust, a change in mood or behaviors upon being placed in a nursing home is normal.

- Trust the nursing home. If you don't, find a different one.

- Keep up-to-date on your care. Know how you are progressing in therapy and when you may be discharged. Understand your medical conditions and treatments. Make sure you are getting proper testing and medication and medical follow-up. Use the nursing home record described below.

NURSING HOME RECORD

Skilled nursing home care is very goal directed. When it is over, the patient will have to make a decision: stay at the nursing home, return home, or go to some other living arrangement. Tracking your care will empower you to partner with the nursing home, ensuring that you will be discharged in a timely fashion. Some nursing homes keep patients at the facility as long as they can in order to maximize reimbursement.

The personal nursing home record (found in Appendix B) allows you to track your care to prevent staying any longer than necessary. The record requires you to fill out information on your health care providers so you know how to contact them. Key personnel you need to know include the nurse in charge of your unit; the director of nursing; the physical, occupational, and speech therapist; and the doctor overseeing your care. It is also important you have a basic understanding of the plan of care for the therapy services. Therapists are required to develop a plan of care and an estimated time you will be in the therapy. Make sure you discuss with each therapist his or her plan so it can be recorded on the form.

If you are receiving skilled nursing care, make sure you understand your goals. For example, if you are receiving intravenous antibiotics for a wound infection, you should know for how long and when you are to follow up with the doctor. While those who are placed in a nursing home under therapy services are discharged when therapy is maximized, those who are under a skilled nursing benefit are discharged when the doctor feels skilled nursing care is no longer needed. Understanding the plan and when you are to see the doctor is vital.

CHAPTER 7

MEDICINES: DO I NEED ALL OF THESE MEDICINES?

*F*ifty-four-year-old John goes to his doctor and complains of heartburn. *The doctor gives John a drug called a proton pump inhibitor and quickly pushes him out the door. John is already on five medications and cannot afford another. He does not fill the prescription and his signs and symptoms get worse.*

Other treatment options are available that do not require medication. Lifestyle changes can have a profound effect in the treatment of heartburn. Teaching a patient about lifestyle changes is much more time intensive than prescribing a drug, and many doctors find it easier to prescribe medications.

John needs not only knowledge but also communication skills to avoid being prescribed another medicine. This is a situation where the patient needs to voice an active opinion to get his desired outcome. Medications are often very effective at treating disease, but they are not without risk. Medications have the potential to produce side effects, interact with other medicines, and drain your bank account.

This frequently happens in health care. John was prescribed an appropriate medication, but there were other options available. Applying the communication skills learned in this chapter will allow the reader to partner with his or her doctor to help make decisions. Without collaboration, patients will be doing what is most convenient for the doctor, not necessarily what is best for the patient.

Older Americans are overexposed to inappropriate drugs, which leads to many problems. According to the Merck Manuel, community dwelling patients over sixty-five are on an average of four to five prescriptions and one to two over-the-counter medicines. The average nursing home resident is on seven to eight prescription medicines.[1] Not only can all this medicine harm your body, it can also put a dent in your pocketbook. Five drugs can cost six thousand dollars annually; even those with insurance may face a thousand dollars a year in out-of-pocket expenses.

Why So Many Drugs?

Prescribing a medicine is an easier solution than spending time teaching the patient about lifestyle changes. Diabetes, high blood pressure, and high cholesterol are examples of diseases that can be treated with lifestyle interventions.

While lifestyle interventions are great treatment options for many diseases, they require work by both patient and physician. Many patients are unsuccessful at incorporating them into their lives. It also takes doctors a lot of time to teach these techniques, and many feel that their efforts are fruitless. A doctor may argue, "Why should I spend all that time teaching about a lifestyle change that a person will likely not comply with when I could prescribe a drug that would do the same thing and take up less of my time?"

In today's health care climate, patients see multiple specialists. While this helps assure that each condition is being treated appropriately, it often leads to a dilemma that health care professionals call polypharmacy. Polypharmacy is a situation where individuals are on multiple medicines that may be duplicate medications or ones that interact with one another. Generally speaking, the more specialists a patient sees, the more medicines he or she is going to be on. Many doctors feel the need to do something about any complaints a patient has. At times this is justified, but every complaint does not need a medicine.

Patients also typically come out of the hospital on more medications than when they went in, and have no idea why. For example, when a patient is in the hospital they are often placed on something to protect his or her stomach from ulcers. These medications are sometimes not stopped and are carried on to the discharge papers. These drugs are often not needed on a long-term basis and could safely be stopped, but are often not stopped.

Drug companies are partly responsible for the overprescribing of medicine. The companies spend billions of dollars a year advertising their drugs. Many continuing education conferences and programs sponsored by drug companies do a great job of promoting treatment of a specific disease or symptom with a specific medication. Conferences sponsored by drug companies are very popular because they often provide gifts and food for attendees. Few continuing education conferences focus on lifestyle changes to heal the body. Who would sponsor such a conference?

Consumer advertising raises public awareness about the effectiveness of medication. When the consumer understands a drug can treat a certain condition, he or she is likely to ask the doctor for it. If there were more advertisements about controlling cholesterol, blood pressure, and diabetes with exercise, would more patients be asking the doctor about these as treatment options for his or her disease?

ADVERSE DRUG REACTIONS: WHY THEY INCREASE WITH AGE

It is estimated that 1.5 million people are admitted to the hospital and 100,000 deaths occur every year because of adverse drug reactions.[2]

Age-related changes increase the risk. The kidneys function less effectively as one ages. Doses that could be handled in a twenty year old will not be excreted in an older individual and will build up the body, leading to increased risk of toxicity. The liver, which also breaks down many drugs, tends to lose function with age. In addition to the age changes, many disease processes are more common in the older population that decrease organ function and lead to a more difficult time metabolizing medicines.

Normal age-related changes increase the risk for adverse drug reaction. Total body water is decreased in the older population, so these people are at increased risk of dehydration if they have high blood pressure and are treated with a diuretic, which depletes the body of water.

The amount of protein in the blood decreases as one ages. One of protein's jobs is to binds certain medications, most notably seizure medicines and blood thinners. Less protein in the blood translates to more active medication in any given dose, making patients are more prone to toxic levels.

Also, older individuals have a decreased ability to absorb medicine due to changes in the gastrointestinal tract.

MEDICATION ERRORS

The causes of medication errors are varied. In the outpatient setting, a common error is the pharmacist filling the wrong prescription due to the inability to read the physician's handwriting. Patients who do not understand instructions are another cause of error. Communication with the doctor and pharmacist can reduce errors in the outpatient setting.

It is essential that your doctor communicates with you about the drug he or she is prescribing. A critical step in reducing errors is utilizing the doctor visit forms in Appendix B. Take notes on any new drug prescribed. In addition, use the questions outlined at the end of this chapter (Table 6.2) when you are prescribed a new drug. If you have good notes on what the doctor prescribed, you will be able to question the pharmacy if any inconsistency is noted.

In the hospital, errors often result from lack of attention rather than lack of knowledge. The nursing staff is often overworked and makes errors in administering medicine. Another cause of hospital errors is the failure to get an accurate history from the patient. The doctor performing the initial work-up may not get an accurate list of the medications the patient takes, for example.

Using the hospital form in Appendix B will reduce the risk of getting an incorrect medication. Keeping your personal hospital chart next to your bed helps to see that you receive only medications that are meant for you. In addition, presenting an accurate medical history and list of medications you are currently on when you enter the hospital reduces the risk of drug errors.

SIDE EFFECTS

All medicines have side effects, and many side effects are known and considered normal. Some medicines have more side effects than others. Some side effects subside when the patient gets used to the drug while others persist indefinitely. Some side effects are easy to spot such as diarrhea and others are subtler, such as fatigue.

Side effects vary by drug and can range from a mild inconvenience to life threatening. Common side effects include: fatigue, diarrhea, constipation, nausea, vomiting, decreased appetite, memory impairment, and kidney dysfunction. Life-threatening side effects include abnormal heart rhythms and lung damage. It is important to discuss side effects with your doctor when you are being placed on a new drug. When you start a new drug, you will typically have a follow-up appointment with your doctor. This is the time to discuss and report side effects.

Knowing about the new drug is a key feature to health care responsibility. Understanding why the drug is taken, its side effects, and follow-up needed is essential. Always ask the questions listed at the end of this chapter (Table 6-2) when you are prescribed a new drug.

DRUG INTERACTIONS

Drug interactions are negative effects resulting from the mixing of two or more medications. Drugs can intensify or blunt the desired effect of another medication. For example, patients on a blood thinner called coumadin need to have tight control of the blood level, requiring frequent laboratory evaluation to assure the drug is therapeutic. The addition of an antibiotic has the potential to increase or decrease the amount of drug in the blood, placing the patient at elevated risk for bleeding complications if levels become too high or risk of clots if levels are too low. Individual variation is common with drug interactions.

Older adults are on more medicines and therefore have an increased risk of drug interactions. Medical science lacks extensive research on drug interactions, especially when patients are on more than two or three drugs.

Whenever you are started on a new drug, talk to the doctor and pharmacist about any potential interactions. Pharmacists may have a better idea of the interactions present because they have computer programs available to help sort out complicated drug regimes.

COMPLICATIONS

Complications are adverse events from drugs that cannot be classified as a side effect, interaction, or error. A bacterial infection causing severe diarrhea secondary to antibiotic therapy, called Clostridium difficile (also known as C. Diff.), is one common complication. Clostridium difficile is a bacterium that invades the gastrointestinal tract, causing severe diarrhea. Another complication is addiction to drugs, especially sedatives and painkillers. Drugs are not benign substances;

health care providers need licenses to prescribe them for good reason. With the many potential errors, side effects, drug interactions, and complications, extreme caution must be used when using medication.

New Drugs: They Must Be Better

Drug company representatives do a great job marketing new drugs. I am amazed at how frequently I see physicians put patients on drugs that have just come to the market. These drugs are often prescribed when there is a similar drug that has many years of proven safety and efficacy behind it. It is understandable if a patient has a life-threatening illness and the new drug is the only option, but this is typically not the case.

Be cautious about the use of new drugs. When a new drug is approved, many things are not known about it, such as all side effects and adverse reactions. Question your doctor carefully if he or she prescribes a drug that has been recently approved. Ask why you should use this new drug as opposed to an older, better-studied drug. Your doctor may have good reason to prescribe the new drug, but it is important for him or her to explain why it is being prescribed.

An estimated $2.5 billion was spent on direct to consumer advertising for medicines in 2000.[3] Much of that money is spent on the newer medicines. Between the years of 1975 and 1999, approximately 10 percent of the newly approved drugs were pulled off the market or a serious warning was placed on them after they received Food and Drug Administration (FDA) approval.[4] Many drug problems surface after FDA approval, when a larger number of patients are placed on the drug.

TABLE 6-1
QUESTIONS TO ASK ABOUT NEW DRUGS

- What evidence is there that this drug is better than a more established drug?

- Has evidence been published in a reputable journal?

- Did your information come from a peer-reviewed journal or from a drug rep?

- Do you have any financial ties to the company that makes this drug?

- Are you paid to put me on this drug, for example through a drug study?

COMPLIANCE

Medicines are expensive. Some older patients have to choose between taking medicine and eating. It is not unusual for a patient to get a prescription for a new drug at the doctor's office and then to be unable to afford to fill the prescription. This can result in progression of disease, resulting in the doctor prescribing another medicine that the patient cannot afford.

If you are unable to take the medicine for any reason, tell your doctor. Other solutions often exist, but they cannot be implemented if the doctor thinks you are taking the drug.

OVER-THE-COUNTER MEDICINES

Over-the-counter (OTC) medicines are generally safe when taken by healthy adults. These drugs are not without risk, especially in the older adult with other health problems. Some OTC medicines interact with prescription medicines. Pharmacists, if they are familiar with your medical history, can help guide you to safe and effective OTC medicines.

Some OTC drugs need to be used with special caution. Acetaminophen (Tylenol) needs to be used in moderation in patients who drink alcohol on a regular basis or have liver disease. The combination of acetaminophen and alcohol can lead to liver damage. Another potential complication includes combining ibuprofen (Advil, Motrin) or Naproxen (Aleve) with alcohol, due to the potential for a stomach bleed. Patients who are on warfarin (coumadin) need to use caution when taking any OTC. Medicines have a tendency to interact with warfarin causing either drug levels going too high and putting you at risk for bleeding or lowering drug levels and putting you at risk for developing a blood clot.

Many remedies for colds have the potential for side effects. Most people do not think twice about taking a cold remedy but they can be very dangerous. Two popular ingredients in cold remedies—decongestants, which help to reduce nasal congestion, and antihistamines, which can decrease sneezing and dry up watery eyes or a runny nose—have potentially fatal side effects. Decongestants have the potential to increase blood pressure. Antihistamines have the potential to cause increased confusion, constipation, retention of urine, and dry mouth.

Never exceed the recommended dose of over-the-counter medicine.

WHEN STARTING A NEW MEDICINE ASK NUMEROUS QUESTIONS.

It is important that you have a complete understanding of your medicines. Medicines are prescribes for multiple reasons after careful consideration from your health care provider. Below (Table 6-2) is a list of questions that you should know about each medicine.

TABLE 6-2
QUESTIONS TO ASK ABOUT EACH MEDICATION

- What is this medicine for?

- Does my age affect the dose needed to treat me properly?

- Are there any restrictions with this drug? For example, should I not drive after taking the drug?

- How will it help me? How will I know if it is working?

- When should I take the medicine? In the morning? At night?

- Should I take the medicine with food or on an empty stomach?

- What are the common side effects? Are the benefits of this drug worth the side effects and drug interaction?

- Are there any necessary follow-ups by exam or laboratory evaluation for monitoring this medicine?

- How long will I need to take this medicine? Will I be on this drug for life?

- How much does it cost? Are there any cheaper alternatives to this medicine? Is there a generic version that has equal effectiveness?

- Can this medicine interact with any of my other medicines?

- How long has this medicine been on the market?

- Are there any severe risks with this medicine?

- What should I do if I miss a dose?

- Can I drink alcohol while on this medicine?

AN EXAMPLE OF POLYPHARMACY

Diabetes, a condition where the body is unable to use insulin or does not make enough insulin, requires several medications to manage. This includes not only diabetes itself but also the multiple other medical conditions associated with diabetes such as high blood pressure, heart disease, kidney failure, nerve damage, erectile dysfunction, and stroke. It is not uncommon for a diabetic patient to be on over ten medications a day.

Fewer complications of diabetes occur when an individual has tight control over his or her blood sugar. Five oral classes of diabetes medicines, two new injectable medications, and insulin are used to manage diabetes. It is not uncommon for a diabetic to be on two pills for control of the blood sugar, and many patients are on three. In addition to controlling blood sugar, tight control of blood pressure is another essential element in reducing complications of diabetes. Angiotensin converting enzyme inhibitors or angiotensin receptor blockers, two types of blood pressure medicines, are recommended to control blood pressure due to their ability to limit the damage that diabetes does to the kidneys. Unfortunately, most diabetics are unable to control blood pressure to recommended ranges on just one blood pressure medicine. Many need at least two, and some diabetics take up to five medicines to achieve optimal blood pressure readings. Diabetics are at high risk for heart disease, and there are strict recommendations on control of cholesterol. Many diabetics are unable to control their cholesterol with diet and lifestyle changes alone, and many are on cholesterol-lowering medicine. And, the American Diabetic Association recommends that all diabetics be placed on an aspirin.

Neuropathic pain, a burning pain that results from damage that the high sugar levels do to the nerves, is a common complication of diabetes and often requires medication. Some diabetics need more than one type of pain medicine to control the neuropathic pain. Diabetic men are at high risk for erectile dysfunction that is a condition commonly treated with another pill such as sildenafil (Viagra). Gastroparesis, a slowing of food through the stomach, results from damage to the nerves of the gastrointestinal tract. This condition is commonly treated with the medication metoclopramide (Reglan).

Most diabetics need at least six medicines just to control one disease process, which does not account for other medicines needed to control other disease states.

Some diabetic patients take over 20 pills a day. When diabetics are on multiple medications it is sometimes impossible to predict how they are going to interact with on another.

SUMMARY

It is important that you take an active role in monitoring your medicines. You are at greatest risk when a new medicine is started or when you enter a new health care system. When you are admitted to the hospital or a nursing home, caution must be used to assure you are receiving the proper medications.

HEALTH RESPONSIBILITY: WHAT CAN YOU DO?

1. Keep a written list of all your medicines including the names, doses, and why they were prescribed. Use the form in Appendix A. This medication list will be part of your personal health care record.

2. Prepare your medications each week in a pill storage container that can be purchased at any drug store. Pill containers can be purchased with a compartment for each day or multiple compartments for each day. Place the drug container in an easily accessible location. Use the daily medication list form in Appendix A. Keep this list next to your pill container box.

3. Keep a medication list at your bedside when you are in hospital to assure you are receiving the proper medicines. This is part of your hospital chart shown in Appendix B.

4. Keep a list of medicines previously prescribed. Patients are often tried on medicine that is ineffective or whose side effects were too great to warrant its continued use. Doctors who are seeing the patient for the first time need to know what medicines the patient used in the past and the reason a certain drug was discontinued. Some doctors treat patients as chemistry experiments. Older patients often have a long medical history behind them, and knowing that history will help cut down on much of the guesswork in prescribing medications. Utilize

the form in Appendix A and make it part of your personal medical record.

5. Ask questions. Understand why you are on each medication and make sure your doctor gives you all the information. Whenever starting a new medicine, ask the questions listed in table 6-2.

6. Make sure there is a reason for taking each of your medicines. This may seem silly, but some patients are on medications even though neither doctor nor patient is sure why.

7. Whenever you are started on a new medicine, ask your pharmacist about drug interactions. Drug interactions are sometimes not considered by doctors when prescribing medicine. Your pharmacist should know your medical history and allergies. The pharmacist also can help guide you to taking proper OTC medications.

8. Take notes when a new medication is prescribed.

9. Take your medical record, including your medication list, when you are admitted to the hospital.

10. Do not pay attention to direct to consumer advertising. It is set up to sway your thinking.

11. Take your personal health care record to the pharmacy.

SECTION 3

HEALTH PROMOTION/DISEASE PREVENTION

CHAPTER 8

Preventative Health Care

*F*ifty-five-year-old Luke had a strong family history of heart disease. His father died of a heart attack at the age of fifty-three and his mother died after complications of a stroke at fifty-eight. He has one brother who was a diabetic and had one silent heart attack at forty-eight. His brother died at sixty-one from complication of diabetes. Luke is five-foot-eight and 170 pounds when he first sees his doctor. His blood pressure, cholesterol, and lab work are all normal.

Based on his strong family history, Luke is encouraged by his primary care physician to maintain a healthy weight, exercise regularly, eat healthy, have annual physical exams, and take one aspirin a day.

Luke returns to his primary care doctor next year, weighing 198 pounds. His blood pressure is 150/94 mmHg and his heart rate is 94. His total cholesterol is 268 mg/dl, his bad cholesterol 175 mg/dl, good cholesterol 30 mg/dl, and triglycerides 315 mg/dl. His fasting blood sugar is 122 mg. Based on these lab readings, he is diagnosed with high blood pressure, high cholesterol, obesity, and glucose intolerance.

Luke's doctor encourages him to lose weight, start an exercise program, and start living better. He is also placed on a blood pressure pill called metoprolol extended release and a cholesterol pill called atorvastatin and is told to continue with the daily aspirin. These interventions have a goal of preventing or delaying a significant cardiac event.

Luke does reasonably well on the medical plan and complies with his disease management. He engages in a regular exercise program and begins a heart-healthy diet. The next year, Luke's weight is back down to 170 pounds, his blood pressure and cholesterol are well controlled, and he is able to come off his blood pressure and cholesterol pills.

Luke maintains this pattern for five years, but has a heart attack at sixty-two. He is placed back on his cholesterol and blood pressure pills. He is enrolled in a cardiac rehabilitation program and he continues to exercise, eat well, and take his medicine. Because of his regular exercise program, Luke feels good and has a good quality of life.

At the age of seventy-six, Luke developed a major stroke and dies six months later. While the ultimate outcome was still death, he outlived everyone in his family. He was at high risk for developing cardiovascular disease. Living a healthy lifestyle by eating well, exercising, and having regular doctor appointments not only extended the quantity of his life but also improved the quality of his life.

Chronic disease kills. Fortunately, chronic disease can be prevented or delayed. Preventative health care is a broad term that incorporates a variety of activities that prevents problems before they occur or catches them before they do too much damage to the body. Disease states can be treated more easily if they are detected early. Examples of preventative health care include exercise, good nutrition, stopping or not starting smoking, minimizing alcohol intake, receiving recommended immunizations, and having recommended health screenings.

Everyone will die; but approximately 40 percent of deaths are related to smoking, bad diet, lack of exercise and alcohol intake. Many preventative health activities you can do on your own, but several activities require partnering with your health care provider. For example, exercise is something you need to motivate yourself to do every day; you cannot rely on your doctor to do it for you. But exercise sometimes requires clearance and certain restrictions from the doctor.

National organizations have set up guidelines for preventative health care services. The preventative health care worksheet, found in Appendix A, provides some general guidelines.

Preventative health care is underutilized in the United States for a variety of reasons. Individuals often lack proper education about its importance or what it entails.

Developing a partnership with a primary care doctor is an important first step in preventative medicine. This is best accomplished if you have your health care information organized. Step three of the personal health record in Chapter 11 provides a framework for recording and tracking preventative health care.

WHAT YOU NEED TO KNOW

Do not assume that your doctor will remember to discuss, recommend, or provide all the necessary measures to practice good preventive health care. While some doctors are better at this than others, most doctors simply have too many patients and too little time to do a complete job at preventative medicine. You need to take responsibility. The next section discusses the three main components of preventative health care: healthy lifestyle, health screenings, and immunizations.

HEALTHY LIFESTYLE

Living a healthy lifestyle is one of the most cost-effective, underutilized ways to prevent the development or progression of chronic disease. Living a healthy lifestyle in the American culture where a fast-food restaurant is on almost every corner and it is glamorous to smoke and drink is a challenging prospect.

Developing a healthy lifestyle can be extremely difficult. It involves changing habits of many years. Changing the diet to incorporate fruits, vegetables, and lean meats can be very difficult. Finding sixty extra minutes in the day to incorporate an exercise program may involve major lifestyle shifts.

Many older adults are set in their ways, and it can be difficult to dissuade their patterns developed sixty or more years ago. Many older adults feel that major changes limit the amount of enjoyment they will get from life. This could not be further from the truth; lifestyle changes not only prolong life, but also improve the quality of life. Healthy lifestyle is the number one step to becoming functionally younger.

Lack of knowledge is a common barrier to practicing preventative health care. The five- to ten-minute office visit you have with your doctor is not enough time to learn about preventative health care. The office visit is a time to get limited specific information about healthy lifestyles.

Two major topics in healthy lifestyle, exercise and nutrition, will be discussed at length in the next chapters.

Smoking is one of the worst things you can do for your health. Smoking is associated with diseases including heart disease, stroke, emphysema, and multiple types of cancer. Quitting smoking is one of the most important steps you can take to improve quality and quantity of life.

Experts report alcohol in moderation can have beneficial effects on health. Excessive alcohol can have multiple negative effects, including liver damage, stomach problems, and problems with balance, leading to falls and fractures. Moderate alcohol consumption, which is defined as one drink per day for women and two drinks per day for men, may protect the heart and raise HDL or good cholesterol.

Injury prevention is a broad category that can improve quantity of life. Activities associated with injury prevention include wearing a seatbelt, using smoke detectors/carbon monoxide detectors, conducting home safety evaluations, and setting hot water heaters to 130 degrees or below.

Health Screenings

Health screenings are not meant to pick up every disease possible, but to catch common diseases that when detected early can be cured or their complications significantly limited. It is important to take responsibility for seeing that you receive the proper screening tests. Some common diseases for which you should be screened are high blood pressure; high cholesterol; osteoporosis; diabetes; dementia; depression, hyper or hypothyroidism; and breast, prostate, colon, and cervical cancer as well as vision and hearing problems. Insurance companies will only pay for screening at certain intervals and at certain ages.

Your annual appointment is the time to discuss preventative health care needs. Appendix B has a form that should be filled out prior to the visit. The three-page annual form concludes with questions regarding good preventative health.

Review the preventative health care worksheet in Appendix A. If you are not within the recommended guidelines, ask your provider about that preventative activity. After you have a test, record on this form when the testing was performed and any comments that your doctor makes.

PREVENTATIVE HEALTH CARE WORKSHEET

This worksheet in Appendix A summarizes health screenings. Depending on your overall health status, there will be some variation to the type and frequency of screenings. Diabetics, for example, require specialized testing to detect early complications of the disease. Some people may need more frequent or less frequent evaluations. It is important to talk with your health care provider about each of the items on the form—communication is the key!

EXAMS

Annual exams by your health care provider should include a breast and pelvic exam if you are a female and a prostate evaluation if you are a male. The annual exam is the critical element to assuring good preventative health care.

Dental health is important to overall health. Complications of poor dental health include malnutrition and weight loss. Recommendations for good preventative health include dental visits every six to twelve months, brushing and flossing after each meal, not smoking or chewing tobacco, and limiting concentrated sweets.

Regular eye exams after the age of fifty are a key component to good preventative health care. An eye doctor should examine the eyes every one to three years. Speak with your primary doctor and eye doctor about your recommended frequency.

The incidence of eye diseases—specifically, glaucoma, cataracts, or macular degeneration—is much higher in the older population. Glaucoma can cause blindness but can be prevented or delayed if it is caught early. Risk factors for glaucoma include severe nearsightedness, family history of glaucoma, diabetes, black race, or age (over sixty-five). Be sure to tell your doctor if you are having trouble with your vision.

Those with certain medical conditions are at risk for more problems with the eyes. Those with diabetes need frequent eye exams as a condition called diabetic retinopathy can result in blindness.

A hearing screen by your health care provider should be done on an annual basis after the age of fifty. Common symptoms of hearing loss include turning the television up, difficulty hearing in a crowded room, or difficulty hearing normal conversation. This is a simple office test where the primary care provider evaluates your ability to hear a whispered voice or the sound of her rubbing her fingers together. If this test is deemed abnormal, more extensive testing may be indicated.

Diagnostic Tests

Diagnostic tests are available for most disease processes. This section looks at recommended diagnostic tests for common diseases that can be detected and have a profound impact of quality and quantity of life.

Hypertension, better known as high blood pressure, is significantly correlated with many chronic diseases and should be screened for at least annually. For those with a history of high blood pressure, it may be checked once a month or once a week. For those who are getting medications adjusted, it may be checked daily.

Bone density tests—the most common is called dual-energy X-ray absorptiometry (DEXA)—detect osteoporosis, a thinning of the bones that increases the risk of fracture. These tests should be performed as screening at least once in females over the age of sixty-five and in high-risk individuals at sixty. High-risk men are also candidates for testing.

Breast, colon, and prostate cancer all can be screened for and treated successfully if caught early. There are a number of tests that screen for colon cancer. The simplest and the first line test is checking for blood in stool, and this should done annually. Unfortunately, there are many false positive results associated with this test. This leads to anxiety in the patients and needs further, more invasive testing such as sigmoidoscopy (a shorter scope to look at the colon) or colonoscopy (a longer scope to look at the colon). Sigmoidoscopy is recommended every five years after fifty and colonoscopy is recommended every ten years after fifty. Colonoscopy may be recommended if you are found to have blood in your stool.

Mammograms, the breast cancer screening, generally should be performed every one to two years in females. Discuss with your doctor about the frequency of screening for your individual case.

One-time abdominal aortic aneurysm screening by ultrasound is recommended for men age sixty-five to seventy-five who have ever smoked. Abdominal aortic aneurysm is a weakening of the major blood vessel coming off the heart. If this vessel bursts, it is typically fatal. Evidence has shown that smokers are at increased risk for weakening of this blood vessel. A simple ultrasound can detect this weakening so that intervention can be implemented before it bursts. The one caveat to this test is that it may not be covered by insurance, so talk to your health care provider about this issue.

Peripheral artery disease (PAD) is a blockage of the arteries in the legs. This disease process can lead to nonhealing wounds, leg pain, and even amputation. Screening for PAD is performed with the use of an ankle to brachial index (ABI). This is the ratio of systolic (the top number) blood pressure in the lower extremity divided by the pressure in the arm. When the number is above 0.9, it is considered normal. When the ratio is less than 0.5 one is considered to have severe PAD. Everyone over the age of seventy should be screened, and those between fifty and sixty-nine should be screened if they have any risk factors such as smoking, diabetes, established heart disease, high blood pressure, or high cholesterol.

Tuberculosis (TB), an infection that affects the lungs, can be passed from one person to another and is treated more easily if caught early. A tuberculosis screen is recommended every one to three years for high-risk people. High-risk individuals include those who have been in contact with someone who has TB; live in very crowed conditions; recently arrived from Africa, Asia, or Central or South America; or have kidney failure, diabetes, human immunodeficiency virus, alcoholism, or a history of using intravenous drugs.

Certain testing modalities are worth discussing with your doctor. Electrocardiogram (EKG) is a tracing of the electrical pattern of the heart. Those over the age of fifty (or younger if there is a family or personal history of heart disease) should talk to their doctor about having one. EKGs detect lack of blood flow to certain areas of the heart, an enlarged heart, and any electrical abnormalities. The appearance of the EKG can vary from person to person, so having a tracing before problems arise may help the doctor determine the degree of abnormality when the patient develops problem such as chest pain. Some resistance will be met to the routine use of EKGs on patients who are not having problems. If your doctor does not think it is necessary to have one, that is reasonable.

Chest X-rays are not recommended as a screening test by any national organization, but if you are a smoker it may be helpful as a baseline. Again this will be met with resistance by some doctors and insurance companies, but it is worth discussing.

BLOOD TESTS

Basic blood tests such as a complete blood count (CBC), kidney function test, and electrolyte testing may be done annually to once every few years. No national recommendations exist for these tests, and the amount of testing will vary depending on your other disease states and risk factors. If you had not had these tests evaluated in the past three years, ask your doctor if they should be run.

The thyroid should be checked once at the age of thirty-five and then every five years. If you are being treated for thyroid disease, have a family history of thyroid disease, or have high cholesterol, you may need to be tested more frequently.

Diabetes screens should be done annually in high-risk patients including those who are obese or have high cholesterol, high blood pressure, or a family history of diabetes. Others should be tested at age forty-five and then every three years. The simplest screen and most common way to look for diabetes includes looking at your blood sugar level after an eight-hour fast.

Cholesterol testing including total cholesterol, low-density lipoprotein (LDL), high density lipoprotein (HDL), and triglycerides. High cholesterol is a common precursor of heart disease, the number one killer of Americans. Treating cholesterol can significantly reduce your risk for heart disease and stroke. A screening should be done in the thirties and then as directed by your health care provider, often every five years in those who do not have cholesterol problems and annually in those who do.

Prostate specific antigens (PSA) is a blood test that looks at the amount of protein given off by the prostate gland. Prostate cancer may be indicated if levels are elevated. This blood test, in combination with a rectal exam, is the main way to screen for prostate cancer. The PSA and a rectal exam should be done annually after the age of fifty, and earlier if you are at high risk for prostate cancer and have a life expectancy of greater than ten years. High-risk individuals for prostate cancer include those who have a family history of prostate cancer or who are black.

There is some risk with this test. There is a high false positive result rate. This means that many men without prostate cancer will have abnormal results on this test, requiring further intervention. These men will need to go through a biopsy to rule out disease that is not there. This will not only cost a lot of money but cause discomfort. Conversely, a normal or even low level does not rule out prostate cancer.

IMMUNIZATION

Vaccinations are used to prevent disease, decrease the severity of disease, and decrease death. Most immunizations are given during the developmental years, but there are some immunizations that are given to older adults. Important vaccinations in older adults include the influenza, pneumococcal, and tetanus/diphtheria vaccines.

There are other immunizations that may be needed. They include immunization against hepatitis A & B. Hepatitis A immunization may be needed in those with diseases of the blood or liver, who travel to areas that have high rates of hepatitis A, or who have sex with more than one person. Hepatitis B immunization may be needed in the older adult who is receiving hemodialysis or those who are exposed to blood products, inject drugs intravenously, have sex with more than one partner, or have a sexually transmitted disease. Immunization against mumps, measles, and rubella (MMR) may be needed in people born after 1957 who have not had two immunizations with MMR or documented immunity to the diseases. Individuals may also benefit from a varicella vaccine (chickenpox/shingles vaccine) if there is no history of disease. This may decrease the risk of developing shingles.

A tetanus/diphtheria booster should be given every ten years. Tetanus is a bacterium that enters the skin and affects the central nervous system, resulting in difficulty swallowing, drooling, fever, irritability, convulsions, respiratory or cardiac arrest, and death. Diphtheria, a respiratory disease that is spread by coughing or sneezing, can be fatal.

Influenza or flu can be deadly in the older population and immunization is recommended in patients over the age of fifty or those with chronic diseases such as diabetes or heart, lung, or kidney disease. Chronic diseases that increase risk of death when inflicted with influenza include lung and heart disease and diabetes. It should not be given to individuals who are allergic to eggs or egg products.

The pneumonia vaccine should be given to everyone over the age of sixty-five. It should also be administered to patients with chronic lung, kidney, heart, or liver disease. The vaccine should also be given to those with diabetes or HIV or who have had their spleen removed. This vaccine does not prevent every strain of pneumonia, but does provide protection against the most common and deadly types. Individuals who get pneumonia after receiving the vaccine tend to get a less severe form. The pneumonia vaccine may lose its effectiveness after five years and patients may benefit from revaccination. Talk with your health care provider.

COUNSELING

Talk to your doctor about the following health topics on an annual basis:

- Exercise

- Diet

- Smoking/tobacco use

- Alcohol

- Drug use

- Breast self-exams

- Seat belts

TABLE 8-1
RECOMMENDED PREVENTIVE TESTING FOR HEALTHY MALES AND FEMALES OVER FIFTY

- Pelvic exam/Pap smear (female): recommendations vary. Paps should be carried out annually in woman ages thirty to seventy; after three negative exams, Pap smears can be done every two to three years; after seventy, Pap smears may not be needed in those who have had normal results for the last ten years.

- Prostate exam/PSA (male): annually after age fifty if life expectancy is greater than ten years.

- Eye exam: every one to three years.

- Dental exam: every six months.

- Mammogram: every one to two years for ages fifty to sixty-nine; every one to three years after three negative tests in those seventy and older.

- DEXA bone density scan: at sixty-five for women or after sixty if high risk; also for high-risk men.

- Blood pressure check: at least every two years.

- Cholesterol level: every five years, more often if cholesterol is high.

- Diabetes screen: every one to three years.

- Colorectal cancer screening

  - Rectal exam annually after forty
  - Colonoscopy every ten years starting at age 50
  - Fecal occult blood test every year after age 50
  - Flexible sigmoidoscopy every five years after age 50

- Vision and hearing screening every year starting at sixty-five

- Dementia and Depression screening every year after sixty to sixty-five years

- Abdominal aortic aneurysm screening (one time) by ultrasonography for men age sixty-five to seventy-five who have ever smoked

- PAD screening in everyone greater than seventy or in those greater than fifty if cardiovascular risk factors are present

Preventative Medicine

Supplements

This section provides a brief overview of supplements that can improve health. Discuss the benefits of each vitamin/medicine listed below with your doctor before taking it.

Calcium intake is important in preventing the development of weak bones or osteoporosis. Weak bones lead to broken bones and disability. The recommended amount of calcium to intake each day is 800-1,500 mg calcium. This can be attained through a healthy, well-balanced diet. Many older adults do not eat a healthy, well-balanced diet and supplementation is needed.

Vitamin D must be taken to assure that calcium is adequately absorbed into the system. Vitamin D should be taken in levels of at least 400-800 IU every day. This level can be attained through drinking vitamin D fortified milk or getting exposure of sun. The skin converts sunlight into vitamin D. Most multivitamins have the recommended amount of vitamin D. Many calcium supplements are combined with vitamin D.

Aspirin has been shown in multiple studies to protect against disease such as cardiovascular events. Certain individuals may not be able to take aspirin due to other medical conditions such as a bleeding ulcer or intolerance. Talk to your doctor. If aspirin is recommended, ask if you should take a baby aspirin, regular dose, and/or enteric coated aspirin.

Antioxidants—vitamins with protective properties—are thought by many to prevent diseases such as cancer and heart disease. Vitamin C and E are supplements that protect against multiple diseases. Studies looked at the effects of vitamins A, C, E and found no strong evidence to advocate or contraindicate their use in the prevention of heart disease or cancer.

The B complex of vitamins is essential for the health of many body systems, including energy production and creation of red blood cells. Many health experts recommend high doses of B vitamins as a way to improve energy, but no hard data prove this is effective. Individuals who are deficient in folic acid and B12 may develop anemia. Low levels of folic acid in the body can increase the levels of an amino acid named homocysteine that is correlated with heart disease.

PREVENTATIVE HEALTH WORKSHEET

There is no effective cookie-cutter approach for preventive screenings and immunizations. Many organizations have guidelines to provide patients and doctors with guidance as to which preventative health care measures are necessary. Guidelines incorporate individual variation based on coexisting diseases, family history, and currently prescribed medications.

Appendix A includes a worksheet to track the tests, exams, screens, immunizations, and counseling that each individual should obtain. This form gives the individual an opportunity to record the dates of preventative testing. This tool allows you to see what you are missing and discuss this with your doctor. As you can see, a lot of testing is needed. It is extremely easy for the physician to miss some of the recommended tests in his rushed ten-minute office visit. This is why it is critical that each individual take responsibility for his or her preventative health care.

Exam: Each individual should have at minimum an annual exam with his or her primary care provider. This exam entails a medical history and physical exam and assures that preventative testing is up to date, medications are reviewed, and any new treatment options are discussed. The exam may entail much more than that, but these are general recommendations.

Diagnostic Testing: Using the health evaluation tracking form, record the dates that tests were carried out and a brief comment about the result. If you are not in compliance with the recommendations listed on the form discuss with your doctor as to why it was not done. Utilize the explanations listed above.

Blood Testing: This form provides some guidelines about what blood testing should be performed.

Screens: There are screening tests that should be done on individuals to look for common diseases.

Immunizations: This worksheet allows you to record the date of the recommended immunizations to assure you are up to date.

Counseling: Each year, your doctor should attempt to inform you about the importance of certain practices that will improve quality and/or quantity of life. There is not time in any office visit to get a full lecture on any one of these topics. The topics listed on the sheet are among the most common topics that can help individuals practice good preventative health care.

Health Care Responsibility

1. Fill out the prevention chart and note where you fall outside the recommended guidelines. Talk to your doctor about which tests you should receive.

2. Ask your doctor:

   • Should I take a multivitamin?

   • Should I take a daily aspirin?

   • Should I take any other supplements and how much? Specifically ask about calcium; vitamin D, A, C, E and selenium; and the B vitamins, folic acid and B12.

CHAPTER 9

EXERCISE

Not exercising can kill you. Poor diet and physical inactivity account for four hundred thousand deaths per year in the United States. Exercise maintains a high quality of life. The aging body goes through numerous changes that lead to disability, and the rates of disability increase in individuals who are inactive.

Tasks that older adults once took for granted become tremendously difficult with aging. For example, bringing the groceries in from the car is a simple task, but with aging it becomes exceedingly difficult. The decrease in strength and endurance that comes with aging can render the older adult less able to handle such routine tasks of daily living. This decline in function is not inevitable. Individuals who regularly exercise can maintain function and continue doing such tasks without difficulty.

Exercise protects against a number of the chronic diseases common to older adults. Diabetes, high blood pressure, abnormal cholesterol levels, and heart disease are positively affected by exercise. Exercise improves strength and ability to function and live independently.

EXERCISE AND ITS BENEFITS

Three types of exercise maintain health and function: aerobic exercise, strength training, and stretching. Aerobic exercise improves the health of the heart, lungs, and circulatory system while preventing, delaying, and treating certain diseases. Strength training improves muscle and bone strength, and reduces the risk of falling. Stretching keeps the muscles loose and prevents injury. Well-balanced exercise programs incorporate all three types.

You do not have to be Arnold Schwarzenegger or Lance Armstrong to benefit from exercise. The amount of exercise necessary to maintain health is different from the amount needed to attain maximum fitness. This chapter teaches what you need to do to maximize health without living at the gym.

Regular exercise helps the heart function better. Specifically, exercise lowers blood pressure, improves cholesterol, reduces strain on the heart, decreases the stickiness of the blood, and improves the clot-dissolving capacity of the blood. This all translates into a lower risk of cardiovascular disease—including heart attack, stroke, and peripheral vascular disease—which is the leading cause of death.

Exercise improves psychological function. It prevents and treats depression and anxiety. It has also been shown to reduce cognitive decline, which is a predecessor of dementia.

Exercise improves the function of the heart and reduces the risk of diseases of the vascular system. Exercise has beneficial effects on blood pressure, cholesterol, blood sugar, and body weight. Improvements on these parameters can have a profound effect on death and disability.

Exercise improves the immune system. It reduces the chances of getting a viral or bacterial illness. It may also decrease the risk of getting cancer, especially colon cancer. Exercises can also help induce sleep.

Aerobic exercise develops endurance and has been shown to delay or prevent many illnesses. It uses large muscle groups to increase the heart and respiratory rate.

Strength training is not just for body builders. It improves functional capacity, increases muscle mass, improves fat burning, and strengthens bones. Strength training involves putting stresses on the muscles thereby forcing the body to adapt and improve its strength. There are a variety of ways to accomplish strength training including free weights, machine weights, and using the weight of your body.

Strength training has benefits that are different from aerobic exercise. Strength exercises increase bone strength, thereby decreasing risk of osteoporosis and broken bones. Strength training also strengthens muscles, which improves functional ability and decreases the risk of falls. Strengthening the back and stomach reduces back pain.

Exercise strengthens bones and reduces the risk of fractures. Weight-bearing exercises such as walking and jogging are better than non-weight-bearing exercises such as swimming and biking at improving bone strength.

Stretching is associated with many benefits. Flexibility is the ability of the limbs to move through a complete range of motion. Flexibility training maintains range of motion that is often lost with the aging process. Poor flexibility is associated with injuries, especially low back injuries. It provides an overall sense of well-being and relaxation.

The greatest benefit of exercise is the maintenance of independence. Exercise prevents declines in functional capacity. Older adults frequently fear being placed in a nursing home because they are unable to care for themselves. Everyone declines physically with age, but those who do not exercise speed up that decline. Without exercise, the muscles shrink and strength decreases.

RISK OF EXERCISE

While exercise is one of the healthiest things you can do to maintain and improve health, there is risk. The risk for a heart attack is increased during an exercise session. Still, those who exercise regularly are at decreased risk for death than nonexercisers.

It is important to discuss starting an exercise program with your doctor. It is rare that you will not be allowed to exercise, but the doctor may want certain precautions taken before an program is initiated. Some individuals need a stress test prior to starting a program, and some individuals should only participate in certain types of exercise.

The muscles and bones are at increased risk in the older individual. Certain precautions must be implemented to prevent problems. A little bit of soreness is normal, but excessive soreness a day or two after exercise indicates that one is training too rigorously. Those individuals who were less active prior to starting an exercise program and those with many medical diseases are at increased risk for soreness and muscle injury. Initiating an exercise program under the supervision of someone trained in working with the older population is advisable. An experienced exercise professional has the ability to prevent injury and make exercise safe and enjoyable.

CHRONIC DISEASES

Chronic disease is not a barrier to exercise. In fact, those with chronic disease should be exercising more. Diseases such as diabetes, heart disease, and high blood pressure can all be treated at least partially with exercise. When you have chronic disease, it is important to talk with your doctor before undertaking an exercise program so precautions can be taken.

When chronic diseases are not controlled adequately or you are having a new onset of an acute illness, exercise should be avoided. Some conditions include chest pain; irregular or fast heartbeat; fever; severe shortness of breath; significant, on-going weight loss; blood clot; infection; hernia; dehydration; new joint swelling or pain; abdominal aortic aneurysm (a weakness in the wall of the heart's major out-going artery); or narrowing of one of the valves of the heart.

EXERCISE PRESCRIPTION

Exercise prescription, the formula that describes how you should exercise, needs to be individualized. To develop a safe and effective exercise plan, work with a certified exercise specialist. Many books provide a more detailed look at the specific exercise prescription. Books written by the American College of Sports Medicine (ACSM) are great texts that provide more detail into the specifics of the exercise prescriptions.

AEROBIC EXERCISE

Aerobic exercise prescriptions can be broken down into frequency, intensity, length, and mode of exercise. This section provides an overview of the components to aerobic exercise. There is no cookie-cutter recipe for exercise prescription. Individuals just starting an exercise program have a different prescription than those who have been exercising for years. Gradually working your way into an exercise program is important to prevent soreness and injury. Working with an exercise physiologist, who specializes in working with older adults, can help in this process.

Frequency

Recommended frequency for aerobic exercise is three to seven times a week. Exercising three times a week with one-day rest between exercise sessions is a reasonable starting goal. After a few weeks, increasing your frequency to four days a week is sensible. Adding one day a week every month assures your body adapts to the demands exercise puts on it without causing undue soreness, injury, or psychological burnout.

Do not overcommit to an exercise program, especially in the beginning. Optimal health is accomplished with frequent exercise. Working up to some form of aerobic exercise every day is a good goal for all to have. Benefits of exercise are maximized with daily or almost daily exercise. While many organizations suggest exercising every day, caution should be applied. Not only does this increase the risk of injury, especially for the novice exerciser, it may cause burnout. Many well meaning people start off exercising six to seven days a week, only to be burned out of exercising within three weeks.

Another key to preventing soreness or injury is a concept called cross-training. Cross-training involves varying the activities that you do. This provides many benefits; not only will it prevent soreness and injury, but it reduces boredom and trains multiple muscle groups.

Intensity

Intensity is a fancy way of saying how hard you exercise. While elite athletes may benefit from intense exercise, moderate exercise is recommended for the general population. Health benefits are maximized and risks minimized with moderate exercise. The old adage "no pain, no gain" does not ring true when it comes to the benefits of exercise.

How can you tell if your exercise is too vigorous? Activity that makes you breathe and sweat hard can be consider vigorous. Exercise that makes you breathe so hard that you cannot carry on a conversation is considered too hard.

The simplest way to measure intensity is to use the talk test. Exercise to the point that your breathing is increased but are able to carry on a conversation without gasping for air. Do not exercise to a point where you cannot carry on a conversation due to excessive exertion.

More scientific methods of measuring intensity that are popular among exercise professionals include using your heart rate. This is done by exercising at a percentage (typically 50-80%) of your maximal heart rate. Determining your maximal heart rate can be difficult in the older adult. A simple formula for determining your maximal heart rate is to subtract your age from 220. For example, if you are sixty years old, your (theoretical) maximal heart rate would be 220-60 or 160 beats a minutes.

Determining maximal heart rate using this method has problems. Individual variation in maximal heart rate is common; not every sixty year old has a maximal heart rate of 160. Medicines can have a profound effect on heart rate. Many blood pressure medications decrease not only blood pressure but heart rate as well. Medicines that produce a lower heart rate also reduce the maximal heart rate, and formulas to predict maximal heart rates are consequently inaccurate. Individuals who really want to use this method to determine intensity should purchase a heart rate monitor. This is a strap that is worn around the chest that transmits the pulse rate to a watch.

The use of treadmill stress test is one way to get an accurate reading of your heart rate range. The test is often done prior to an exercise program to assure that the patient is healthy enough to exercise safely. Stress tests are also used to screen for heart disease.

When individuals have a stress test, the maximal heart rate is attained. This is not a predicted maximal heart rate, but a true maximal heart rate and can be used by the exerciser to determine an accurate training zone. Not all older adults need a treadmill stress test before starting an exercise program.

Those who are confused by the above formulas need not be concerned. While exercising in a specific heart rate range may be the most scientific way of exercising, it is not necessarily the best. Just getting out and moving your body allows you to derive the benefits of exercise.

If you exercise in a setting staffed by well-trained professionals, using the heart rate method will be very valuable. Exercise professions can help you determine your maximal heart rate and the range in which you should be exercising.

My personal belief is that the heart rate method should not be used by older individuals who are new to exercise. Focus on just getting out there and moving. There are too many barriers to exercising, and getting frustrated with trying to track your heart rate is one more barrier that can inhibit your desire to exercise. Certain groups of patients may suffer from using the heart rate method. Those who take medicine that changes the heart rate, have an irregular heart beat, and have a pacemaker will not get accurate intensity readings from the heart rate method.

DURATION

Duration is another key component to the exercise prescription. Start exercising ten to fifteen minutes a day is a logical place to start, adding of five to ten minutes a week. The eventual goal should be to exercise for thirty minutes a day. Exercise hard enough to burn 200 calories of activity on most days of the week. This can be accomplished by walking or jogging two miles. This may not be a realistic goal initially, but should be a long-term goal.

TYPE

The last component is the type of exercise. Aerobic exercise involves increasing the heart rate and breathing rate with exercises using big muscle groups such as the legs. Ideal aerobic exercises include walking, biking, exercise classes, and swimming. Many considerations must be kept in mind when deciding which mode of exercise to choose. Despite many claims that certain exercises are better than other exercises, there is no perfect exercise. Personal preference is an important consideration; exercises that are enjoyable will be complied with much better. Oftentimes, the best exercise is a variety of exercises also known as cross-training.

Cross-training not only alleviates boredom but reduces injury by stressing different muscle groups and joints. Cross-training involves spending a certain amount of time on different aerobic exercises and can be accomplished in a variety of ways. Performing a different mode of exercise each time you have an exercise session is one way. For example, Monday would involve walking on the treadmill for twenty minutes, Wednesday would involve a water aerobic class, and Friday exercise includes riding the stationary bike for thirty minutes. Cross-training could also include different types of exercises at each training session. For example, an exercise session might include ten minutes on the stationary bike, ten minutes on the elliptical trainer, and fifteen minutes walking on the track.

STRENGTH TRAINING

The goal of strength training for health purposes is to improve the quality and quantity of your life. While weight training increases the amount and quality of your muscles, the main purpose of the program is to improve your ability to function in day-to-day life and reduce disease.

Strength training is a little bit more difficult to understand than aerobic training. It is important that you understand some common terms.

- Repetition is one lift. For example, while doing a push-up, the act of touching your chest to the floor from the starting position and returning to the starting position is one repetition.

- Set is a series of repetitions of a given exercise. For example, doing ten push-ups is one set.

- Progressive overload means increasing the amount of work done as strength increases. See the example below for a better understanding of progressive overload.

TABLE 9-1	MONDAY	THURSDAY	MONDAY	THURSDAY	MONDAY
Chest press	30 lbs. 10 times (one set)	30 lbs. 11 times (one set)	30 lbs. 11 times (two sets)	30 lbs. 11 times (two sets)	30 lbs. 12 times (two sets)
Leg press	50 lbs. 12 times (one set)	50 lbs. 13 times (one set)	50 lbs. 14 times (one set)	50 lbs. 15 times (one set)	55lbs. 12 times (one set)
Arm curl	20 lbs. 15 times (one set)	20 lbs. 15 times (two sets)	25 lbs. 10 times (two sets)	25 lbs. 11 times (two sets)	25 lbs. 11 times (two sets) & 10 times (one set)

Safety is a key component. Proper breathing is critical to prevent abnormal rises in blood pressure. The most important thing to remember is to not hold your breath. Breathing out with each exertion and breathing in with the easier part of the lift is one way to assure that you are breathing properly. Prior to weight training, it is important to incorporate a warm-up. Warm-ups include at least five to ten minuets of easy walking with light stretching prior to your session

Strength training prescription is different than the aerobic prescription. While aerobic training is recommended to be done daily or almost daily, strength training for health benefits should be done two to three times a week. There should be at least forty-eight hours rest between each weight training session. Your muscles need time to recover and heal after stressing them with weights, and if you lift weights without 48 hours between sessions, you risk doing more harm than good. Many weightlifters lift five to seven times a week, but unless your goal is to be in a bodybuilding contest this is not necessary. Each weight training session should last fifteen to thirty minutes and include at least one exercise for each major muscle group of the body.

Intensity is a difficult concept to understand when it comes to weight training. No specific weight or formula will tell you how hard you should lift. When starting an exercise program, working with an exercise physiologist can help you pick a weight to tax your muscles without inducing injury. When starting, pick a weight that is light and focus on using proper form to prevent injury. Eventually, choose a weight that provides enough challenge so the last repetition in a set is the last repetition you can do without compromising your form.

Progressive overload, or increasing the amount of work done as strength increases, should be applied to resistance training. Progressive overload not only includes the actual amount of weight placed on the exercise bar but also includes increasing the number of sets or the number of repetitions performed. Progressive overload forces the muscle to gain strength. Use caution when applying progressive overload because increasing resistance can provoke injury. Tracking progress assures you maintain progressive overload. Each time you work out, especially in the beginning, strive to increase either the number of repetitions, the amount of weight, or the number of sets you perform. The result will be progressive overload on the muscles and improved strength.

There will be days when you are not feeling as strong and may not feel up to increasing the amount of work that you do, and that is OK. Listen to your body. Never strain or compromise form to overload; this may result in injury.

There is a science behind the number of repetitions that are done. For general health purposes, choose a weight that allows you to perform eight to fifteen repetitions. Power athletes, such as football players or individuals who throw the shot put, typically lift more weight and do fewer repetitions. Choosing a weight that you can lift only three to six times maximizes strength development, but lifting heavy weights increases risk of injury. Selecting a very light weight and lifting it twenty to one hundred times develops muscular endurance.

Weight training that involves one to two exercises for each major muscle group is sufficient to maximize health benefits. Multiple programs exist with some involving time commitments of hours a day. The goal of good health does not require hours a day of weight training. In fact, it only takes about fifteen to twenty minutes of resistance training three times a week to reap the health benefits of resistance training. Performing at least one exercise per major muscle group is recommended (see table 9-2). Spending time with an exercise physiologist is the best way to assure that you are getting a good program developed for you and to assure you have someone showing you how to perform the exercises safely. Details of a well-designed weight training program are beyond the scope of this book.

When meeting with your exercise physiologist, make sure he/she understands your goals. Many people who meet with exercise professionals want to lose weight and shape their bodies. These are important goals, but you may end up getting a program that will not maximize your time. Many body-shaping programs involve spending hours a week working on smaller muscle groups with less focus on strengthening bones and muscles. Exercising for health requires a specific prescription to strengthen the bones and improve muscle strength to improve functional capacity.

Start low and go slow is an old adage many physicians live by when prescribing medicine to older patients. The same can be said about exercise. Use low weights, lower repetitions, and fewer sets when starting a program with the goal of increasing weight, repetitions, and sets as time passes. This minimizes the risk of injury and decreases the incidence of muscle soreness. One set per exercise is a reasonable starting point with the progression of up to three sets per exercise as a goal.

Machine weights are the best mode of strength training for older adults. Machine weights include brands such as Nautilus, Cybex, and many others. While they are expensive and buying a set is not practical for your home, they can be found at any gym. Machine weights are easier to use and less likely to cause injury than free weights.

KEY POINTS TO STRENGTH TRAINING

- Start low, go slow
- Warm up before and cool down after each weight training session
- Perform movements slowly and under control
- Exercise two to three times a week
- Exercise each major muscle group

- Start with one set per exercise

- Work up to two to three sets per exercise

- Take at least forty-eight hours rest between weight-lifting sessions

- Choose a weight with which you can perform eight to fifteen repetitions

- Incorporate progressive overload

STRETCHING

Each major muscle group in the body should be stretched. Stretch each muscle to a point of minimal discomfort and hold. Each stretch should be held for ten to thirty seconds. Improving flexibility comes with the duration of the stretch, not the intensity of the stretch. Do not stretch your muscles to the extremes; this will increase the risk of injury.

To minimize injury, it is best to stretch a warm muscle. Warming a muscle can be accomplished by performing ten minutes of aerobic exercise (such as walking) prior to stretching. Muscles are like a piece of gum. Imagine a cold piece of gum; if you try to bend it, it will snap. If you take a warm piece of gum and bend it, it will bend nicely.

TABLE 9-2
MAJOR MUSCLE GROUPS

- Chest

- Back

- Quadriceps

- Abdominals

- Lower Back

- Shoulders

- Hamstrings

- Biceps

- Triceps

- Calves

SUMMARY

The benefits of exercise are numerous and should be incorporated into the health care practice of almost every individual. A well-designed exercise program should incorporate aerobic training, strength training, and stretching.

HEALTH CARE RESPONSIBILITY

1. Discuss exercise with your doctor utilizing the questions below. Ask if there are any reasons you should not be exercising or any precautions you need to take.

2. Get moving. Doing something is better than nothing.

3. Work with an exercise professional; at least at first, this is the best way to assure you will not induce injury.

Questions to ask your health care provider

- Should I be exercising?

- What type of exercise should I do? Aerobic, strength, flexibility? (The answer should probably be all of the above.)

- What should be my exercise prescription—frequency, intensity, time, and type?

- Should I have a stress test prior to exercising?

- Are there any precautions I should take?

- Are there any exercises I should not do?

- Do you know of any gyms that cater to older adults or that have certified exercise physiologists?

CHAPTER 10

HEALTHY EATING

A healthy diet maintains a healthy body weight, prevents disease, and minimizes the effects of established disease. There is much confusion about what constitutes good nutrition. Whole books have been written about nutrition but this section looks at some nutritional topics and helps you understand how to practice health care responsibility.

GOALS FOR HEALTH RESPONSIBILITY

- Maintain or attain an ideal body weight.

- Eat a healthy mix of food.

- Limit quantities of "bad" foods.

- Understand how disease affects your nutrition.

OBESITY

America is an obese society. When the human body takes in more energy (in the form of food and drink) than we burn off (in the form of activity and exercise), the body stores that extra energy as fat. Our culture is centered on food. Most social events revolve around food, high-calorie food can be found in most workplaces, and a fast-food restaurant is on almost every corner. While fast food in itself is not the main determinant of obesity, what we choose to eat at fast-food restaurants contributes to obesity. Hamburger, small fries, and a diet soda—a reasonable meal at a fast-food restaurant—comprise about 500 calories. Unfortunately, a more typical meal includes a double cheeseburger, large fries, and a large soda, totaling 1,450 calories. That many calories are enough energy to sustain many individuals for a whole day, not just one meal.

Maintaining an ideal body weight is a primary goal of good nutrition. Obesity has reached epidemic proportions in the United States with approximately 30 percent of the population being classified as obese. There is much debate about the best weight-loss diet; but it all boils down to calories. Consuming more calories than you expend in a day results in weight gain. Consuming fewer calories than you expend results in a weight loss.

Weight loss is slow process. One pound of fat is equivalent to 3,500 calories. This means that losing one pound requires a calorie deficit of 3,500 calories. A diet that consists of cutting 300 calories out of the diet a day combined with an exercise program that burns 200 calories a day (walking two miles) results in a 500 calorie deficit. This produces a one-pound weight loss a week. Continuing on this course, ten pounds of weight will be lost in two and one-half months. This is unacceptable in a society where we want things now.

Body Mass Index

Body mass index is a method used by health care providers to help define risk of body weight. It utilizes a mathematical formula to classify patients as underweight, normal body weight, overweight, and obese. Body mass index is determined by dividing the weight in kilograms by your height in meters squared (see example in Table 10-1).

TABLE 10-1
BODY MASS INDEX

Chris, a sixty-eight-year-old man, weighs 200 pounds or 90.9 kilograms and is 5 feet 9 inches or 1.75 meters tall

To determine his body mass index, use the following formula

Weight in kilograms/(Height in meters x Height in meters)

90.9/(1.75 x 1.75)=29.7

Chris has a body mass index of 29.7, which places him in the overweight category.

Less than 18.5:   Underweight

18.5 - 24.9:   Normal

25 - 29.9:   Overweight

30 or greater: Obese

NEGATIVE IMPACT OF OBESITY

Obesity increases your risk for heart disease, stroke, high blood pressure, and abnormal cholesterol. Abnormal cholesterol is one of the most common disorders associated with obesity. High low-density lipoprotein (bad cholesterol), high triglycerides, and low high-density lipoproteins (good cholesterol) are the main effects of obesity. Obese individual are at increased risk for high blood pressure.

Obesity increases your risk for diabetes. It decreases the body's ability to use insulin (a condition called insulin resistance). Insulin, a hormone produced by the pancreas, is used to help get the sugar that circulates in the blood into cells. Insulin resistance results in high levels of insulin in the blood. Insulin resistance is strongly correlated with abdominal fat as opposed to fat stored in the legs and hips. High levels of insulin and sugar in the blood have toxic effects on many body systems including the eyes, heart, nerves, and kidneys. Insulin resistance is associated with increased risk for blood clotting, which increases the risk of vascular disease including heart attacks and strokes.

Not only does obesity tax the heart and hormonal system, but also it negatively affects other body systems. Excess body weight puts stress on the joints and leads to an increased risk of arthritis. Cancers linked with obesity comprise breast, prostate, colon, endometrial, and gall bladder cancers. Stress incontinence—leaking of urine during sneezing, laughing, or coughing—is associated with obesity.

Weight loss is associated with a decrease in blood pressure, improved insulin sensitivity, increased high-density lipoprotein levels, and decreased triglycerides. Although hard data are lacking, these benefits should translate into improved life expectancy and a better quality of life.

Weight Loss: Diet and Lifestyle Modification

To combat the negative impact of obesity, people need to lose weight or maintain a healthy weight. Weight loss is accomplished through diet and lifestyle modifications. Not everyone needs to lose weight. If your body mass index is in the ideal body range, maintaining that weight along and eating a well-balanced diet are your ticket to maintaining good health.

Maintaining an optimal body weight is not the only factor to good health. Many alcohol abusers have an ideal body weight, but have poor nutritional status. Eating a healthy diet along with maintaining an optimal body weight are keys to staving off illness and preventing functional decline.

How does one lose weight? It is almost impossible to get through the day without seeing a promotion for the newest diet craze. Which plan is most efficacious for weight loss? The answer to this question is not known, but one principle applies: body weight is determined by the balance between the energy put in your body (in the form of food) and the energy that your body uses (in the form of activity). Weight loss can only be accomplished if your intake is less than your output of energy. Decreased energy intake or increasing physical activity or a combination of the two is the only way to accomplish weight loss.

A word on low-carbohydrate diets. Low-carbohydrate diets are a popular diet craze believed to result in weight loss. The question is: Do they work?

Yes, low-carbohydrate diets do work, although many questions remain unanswered, especially with respect to safety and efficacy. Many prominent organizations such as the American Heart Association and the American Diabetes Association caution against the use of these diets. These diets often incorporate high-protein animal foods, which are usually also high in saturated fat; this increases the risk of coronary heart disease, diabetes, stroke, and several types of cancer. Excessive protein intake increases the risk of osteoporosis as well as kidney and liver disorders. Limited long-term data are available on these diets. Caution must be exercised in those who are affected by multiple disease processes.

Energy-restricted diets, regardless of composition, result in weight loss. The majority of studies point to the low-carbohydrate diet as slightly better in its ability to result in weight loss, at least in the first six to twelve months. Interestingly, when study data is combined, low-carbohydrate diets are no more effective than a standard diet at producing long-term weight loss.

The key to weight loss is long-term lifestyle modification. Long term means making changes that last a lifetime not just changes that result in a ten-pound weight loss in the first few weeks (which is mostly just water). Changing your eating and exercise habits by eliminating the junk and eating healthy foods cuts down on calories. Making changes to a healthy diet using the tips below and adding daily or almost daily exercise for the rest of your life is the only way to have long-term weight loss.

Our culture wants things now, but poor health and obesity is something that occurred over the years. Reversing this process will not occur overnight or the even a week or month. It takes a lifetime commitment. Still, you will notice an immediate improvement in the way you feel both physically and mentally.

KEY POINTS

- To lose weight, eat fewer calories than you expend.

- Know your body mass index and your weight goal.

• Utilize the principle in the exercise section and engage in a safe and effective exercise program.

Healthy Diet

Nutritional status has an immense impact on not only maintaining health but on disease progression and patient healing. Good diets incorporate variety and are composed of lots of fruits and vegetables, whole grains, and lean meats. Certain disease states affect the nutritional status of the older individual. A proper balance of carbohydrates, proteins, and fats is a key factor to a healthy diet.

In a country that has an obesity epidemic, it is surprising that malnutrition has such a profound impact. Those with chronic disease, which is very common among the older population, need to avoid malnutrition at all costs.

Carbohydrates should make up a majority of the diet. Carbohydrates are a hot topic in today's nutrition literature. Not all carbohydrates are created equally. Foods that are high in simple carbohydrates including white bread, white rice, ice cream, candy, soda, and jellies are absorbed very quickly and cause rapid rises in blood sugar. Unlike simple carbohydrates, complex carbohydrates are packed with essential vitamins, minerals, and fiber. Complex carbohydrates include whole grain cereals, beans, and many vegetables. The bulk of your diet should be consumed from complex carbohydrates.

Fiber is an essential food element to prevent disease. Twenty to 30 grams of fiber should be consumed every day. Fiber is found in fresh fruits and vegetables, bran cereals, and beans. Eating a diet high in fiber has multiple benefits including preventing constipation, possibly reducing the risk of colon cancer, aiding in weight loss, improving cholesterol readings, and slowing the absorption of sugars.

Protein requirements do not change with the aging process. High-protein diets do not result in any greater weight loss than a moderate protein level. Some experts suggest that a diet high in protein results in more satiety and leads to increased compliance with a low-calorie diet. High levels of protein have the potential to put extra strain on the kidneys. If you are going to partake in a low-carbohydrate diet (typically, they are high in protein), talk to your doctor first.

A diet low in saturated fat is an important consideration. Partially hydrogenated fats, found in margarine, crackers, cookies, doughnuts, and chips, are particularly harmful to the body's cholesterol. Monounsaturated fats, polyunsaturated fats, and omega-3 fats should be substituted for saturated fats. Monounsaturated fats are found in avocados, olives, and peanut oil as well as peanut butter. Polyunsaturated fats are not as healthy as monounsaturated fats but are better than saturated fats and are found in soybean and canola oil. Omega-3 fats are found in certain fish including mackerel, salmon, and albacore tuna.

Water is vital to live. It is recommended that you drink eight, eight-ounce glasses a day. Older individuals are more prone to dehydration, and drinking water is a good way to prevent that. Benefits of drinking water include less constipation, reduction in fluid retention, and flushing the body of unnecessary substances. Filling up either a sixty-four-ounce water jug (or filling a twenty-ounce bottle three times) and drinking it will meet your daily requirement.

Small quantities of bad food are not necessarily harmful. Avoid large quantities of foods high in sugar and empty in calories or high in trans fat and high in saturated fat. Foods high in sugar and empty in calories include candy and regular soft drinks. Trans fat is found in many processed foods such as chips, cookies, and crackers. Saturated fats are found in fatty red meats, butter, and fried food such as french fries.

NUTRITION AND DISEASE

Older Americans have a decreased need for energy, so they need fewer calories but still need plenty of vitamin and minerals. Water is vital to many functions, and it is critical to get plenty of liquids without caffeine. Diets high in fiber help the gastrointestinal tract. Protein is needed to repair body tissue.

While disease prevention is a major benefit of good nutrition, disease states change nutritional needs. The risk of heart disease, the number one killer of Americans, can be reduced with a healthy diet. Saturated fats are associated with heart disease. Healthy food habits will reduce your risk for heart disease by lowering blood pressure, improving cholesterol, lowering body weight, and reducing diabetes.

Hypertension or increased blood pressure can be significantly affected by diet and body weight. High sodium diets are associated with elevated blood pressure. In addition to reducing sodium in your diet, eating a diet high in calcium, magnesium, and potassium can lower your blood pressure.

Cholesterol levels can be improved with weight loss, exercise, and a diet low in saturated fats and high in soluble fiber. Cutting down on saturated fats will reduce your risk of getting cardiovascular diseases such as stroke and heart attacks.

Increasing the amount of fruits and vegetables you eat lowers your risk of getting cancer.

Kidney disease is just one example of a condition that often requires restrictions of certain foods or fluids. Ask your doctor or dietitian if you need to follow a special diet

Diabetes, which affects over eight million Americans, can be significantly altered by nutrition. While genetics load the gun for the development of diabetes, the environment pulls the trigger. Losing weight can result an improvement of blood sugar and blood insulin levels.

The risk of osteoporosis can be reduced by eating a diet high in calcium and vitamin D. Incorporate vitamin D milk, yogurt, cereals, and fortified juices in your diet.

TABLE 10-1				
Foods High in Saturated Fats	Foods High in Calcium	Foods High in Potassium	Foods High in Sodium	Foods High in Magnesium
Butter Cheese Whole Milk Ice Cream	Milk Yogurt Cheese	Potatoes Bananas Meats Poultry	Processed foods Frozen dinners Chips	Peanuts Broccoli Spinach Soybeans
Foods High in Soluble Fiber	Foods High in Cholesterol	Foods High in Trans Fat	Foods High in Omega 3 Fats	
Oats Bran Beans Some cereals Rice	Eggs Butter Liver	Doughnuts Cookies Crackers Margarine	Mackerel Salmon Albacore Tuna	

VITAMIN SUPPLEMENTS

The best way to get the nutrients you need is by eating a balanced, varied, healthy diet. A single multivitamin taken every day assures that you are getting the recommended daily allowance of vitamins and minerals. Mega doses of vitamins are not all based on fact, and many may be harmful. Some supplements may be helpful in certain situations, but others may cause harmful side effects. Before taking supplements of any kind, check with your doctor.

TIPS TO A HEALTHY DIET

• Consume nutrient-dense food and drink.

• Limit the amount of saturated and trans fats, cholesterol, added salt, sugar, and alcohol.

- Unsaturated fats such as vegetable oils are healthier than saturated fats, but should be used in moderation. Trans fats, which are fats found in partially hydrogenated vegetable oils and many packaged baked goods, should be avoided.

- Eat lean cuts of meats with the fat trimmed.

- Fruits and vegetables are packed with substances that provide many health benefits. Eating at least five servings of fruits and/or vegetables may be the most important step to healthy eating.

- When eating dairy, choose nonfat or 1 percent milk. Use cheeses that are nonfat, low-fat or part skim.

- The most important meal of the day is breakfast. People who skip breakfast have lower metabolic rates, which increases your risk to gain weight.

QUESTIONS FOR YOUR DOCTOR

- What is my ideal body weight?

- What is my BMI?

- Would losing weight benefit my health status?

- What is the best way to lose weight?

- Are there any diets that are unsafe for me?

- How do you feel about low-carbohydrate diets?

- Do I need any vitamin supplementation?

- Do I need a multivitamin?

- Do I need to supplement with calcium and vitamin D?

- Do any of my diseases require specific dietary modifications?

- Should I see a registered dietitian for help with my diet?

SECTION 4

PUTTING IT ALL TOGETHER

CHAPTER 11

THE PERSONAL HEALTH CARE RECORD: THE SEVEN STEPS

This book outlined the key components to health care responsibility: knowledge, organization, and communication. You have gained knowledge about the health care system, how to communicate within it, and how to attain optimal preventative health care. This chapter provides a seven-step system to organize your information so it can be easily communicated to any provider.

Health care responsibility is a process that starts with understanding your medical history and ends with receiving great health care. This process involves organizing your history and understanding your future health care needs. It is an ongoing process, requiring an initial investment of time and energy to complete the personal health record. After the record is set up, it is updated at each health care encounter or with any change in care.

This system allows you to become an expert in your personal health care. Maintaining your record permits easy transmission of information to providers and assures you are in line with national recommendations of health care.

Communication is a vital step to good health care. Face to face contact time with providers is limited, and you need to know how to maximize this time. Good communication is partially accomplished by being organized. The personal health record system outlined here improves communication with the health care system.

The doctor visit is a business transaction. This does not mean that you should be unfriendly, but use the time wisely. Maintaining a personal health care record provides a sense of power and assures you are getting appropriate care.

MEDICAL RECORD

It is a vital that every provider has full knowledge of your medical history. Older patients typically have a long medical histories, and being able to transmit this information clearly provides a distinct advantage in getting the best health care.

The personal health record, similar to a medical chart that a physician or health care system would keep on you, helps you receive the best health care possible. With the fragmentation of the health care system, it is important to have all your information in one spot. Maintaining your health record allows you to stay organized and transmit accurate information to your providers.

Your medical record contains items such as doctor's notes, lab work, surgical reports, and radiological exams. Your personal health record contains these things and more. The personal health record assures that all of your health record is stored in one place. No more worrying about whether your primary care doctor received a copy of a lab test or diagnostic procedure; you will have a copy that you can share.

Medical records are often incomplete. If you receive services from another health care provider or health care system, this information is likely not known to your doctor. Communication within the system is not optimal; each individual must take that responsibility upon himself or herself.

TABLE 11-1
THE IMPORTANCE OF MAINTAINING
A PERSONAL HEALTH CARE RECORD

---

1. Provides a concise and complete way to organize complex medical histories

2. Improves communication of health information

3. Increases quality time with providers as less time is required for doctors to extract information

4. Secures more effective and efficient care

5. Allows patients to be partners in their health care

6. Cuts down on unnecessary testing because tests results will be available

7. Assists in reducing medical errors

WHAT YOU SHOULD KEEP:

- Demographic information including your name, address and emergency contacts

- Insurance information

- Social information including marital status, children, employment history, and smoking, alcohol, and drug history

- Immunization history. Most adults over the age of fifty received vaccinations in childhood. It is important to document this. Vaccines that need to be more specifically documented include the influenza vaccine, pneumonia vaccine, and tetanus/diphtheria vaccine.

- Drug and food allergies and your reaction to those substances

- Medical diagnosis and the year each disease was diagnosed

- Surgeries and the year(s) they were performed

- Family history. Report the medical history of your parents, siblings, and children. Record any illness, the date of illness onset, and cause of death and age at death if applicable. If the family member is still alive, record his or her date of birth.

- Hospitalizations, including the dates, diagnoses, and treatments.

- Procedure notes. A copy of the report of all procedures that you have had including but not limited to colonoscopies, stress tests, and biopsies.

- Doctor Lists. Record the names and contact information for all doctors who are currently treating you. This includes your primary care doctor and any medical specialists such as a dentist, eye doctor, chiropractor, or podiatrist.

- Medication lists. The list should include all prescription and over-the-counter drugs that you take routinely or on an as-needed basis. It also is helpful to have a list of all medications that you have taken in the past. This list should include the name of the drug you have taken, when it was taken, and why you are no longer taking it.

- Diagnostic procedures. Include X-rays, CAT scans, MRIs, echocardiograms, electrocardiograms, and ultrasounds. Obtaining a copy of each of these tests helps prevent duplication of testing.

- Lab work

- Advanced Directives. This is a copy of your wishes at the end of life. Completing the form at the end of appendix A assists your providers and loved ones in understanding how best to care for you.

- Preventative health monitoring. Keeping a list of what and when testing is needed assures you are getting all recommended tests.

- Doctor visits

- Chronic disease monitoring

THE SEVEN STEPS

Set up your personal health care record using the worksheets provided in the appendixes. You can make copies of the pages in the appendix to fill in the sections or download the forms from http://www.hcrbooks.com. Get a three-ring binder and seven divider sheets with tabs. Here is a list of the sections you will create:

1. Health History (located in Appendix A)

2. Medications (Appendix A)

3. Preventative Health Care (Appendix A)

4. Diagnostic Testing

   a) Laboratory

   b) Radiology

   c) Procedures

   d) Surgeries

5. Health Care Encounters (Appendix B)

   a) Doctor Visits

   b) Specialty Doctor Visits

   c) Hospitalization/Nursing Home

6. Advanced Directives (Appendix A)

7. Chronic Disease (See http://www.hcrbooks.com for more information on specific forms for the chronic disease section.)

Step One: Health History

The first section is an overview of your health; it includes demographics and a medical history. Use the first form in Appendix A to provide this information.

- Fill in your name, date of birth, sex, height, weight and date you recorded that weight.

- Fill in the name of your primary and secondary health insurance companies and your policy number(s).

- Report your ethnic background on your mother's and father's side if known. For example, Mother—Hispanic/American and Father—Asian/American.

- What is your religious background? For example, Catholic, Hindu, Jehovah's Witness, Muslim, Protestant, etc.

- What is your highest level of education?

- Do you have a living will? Where is it filed?

- Fill in an emergency contact. Pick someone you would want a health care professional to contact in case you are in a serious accident and are unable to speak. Include the person's name, relationship to you, and phone number.

- Fill in the name of the person whom you have chosen to be your power of attorney (if applicable) for health care and where you filed those papers.

- What is/was your occupation? Are you retired? Did you work with any chemicals or hazardous materials during your professional career? Which ones?

- Fill in your marital status: married, single, divorced, widowed, or living with a significant other.

- List your children and their ages.

- What is your living situation? Do you live alone? Who do you live with? Do you live in an apartment, house, condo, nursing home, or assisted living? How many stairs do you have in your home/apartment?

- Indicate whether you are a smoker. If you have stopped, indicate the date you quit. Estimate the number of packs of cigarettes you smoke(d) on an average day. How many years did you smoke? Fill in any other tobacco use, including pipe use or chewing tobacco.

- Have you ever used or do you currently use any recreational drugs such as marijuana, cocaine, or LSD?

- How many drinks do you consume? Write in the number and circle whether you have that number of drinks per day, week, month, or year.

- Have you ever had a blood transfusion? If so, what was the date? Why did you have the transfusion; for example, did you have a bleeding ulcer, cancer or after surgery? What is your blood type?

- When was your last eye exam? Do you wear glasses or contacts?

- When was your last dental exam? Do you wear dentures? Partials? Full? Upper? Lower?

- Do you wear hearing aids? Do you have any hearing problems?

- List the date of your last immunizations.

- List your medication allergies and what happens when you take those medications.

- List all of your medical conditions and the date(s) that you were diagnosed.

- List all of the surgeries that you have had and the date(s) performed.

- List the diseases and the age at diagnosis (if known) that your first-degree relatives have/had, including cause of death and the date of death if applicable. A first-degree relative is defined as a parent, sibling (brother or sister), or child. For example, Mother: High blood pressure diagnosed at 50, diabetes diagnosed at 60, died at 82 from heart attack.

- List all of your hospitalizations including the dates, reasons you were hospitalized, and treatments you received. For example: June/2004: Pneumonia/Antibiotics. Ask your doctor for a copy of the discharge summary to file in your medical record.

- List all the procedures that you have had including colonoscopies, biopsies, angiograms, or endoscopies and the date. Obtain copies for your medical record.

- List all of your doctors utilizing the doctor list form.

STEP TWO: MEDICATION LIST

Next, complete the medication list. It includes the name and dose of each medicine that you are taking as well as the times of the day that you take it and the reason that you are taking it.

In addition, list to the best of your ability medications that you were on in the past. Include the name of the medicine and dose you were on and the date it was started and stopped. Provide a brief explanation. Finally, list any problems or side effects that you had while you were on the medicine.

STEP THREE: PREVENTATIVE HEALTH CARE

Preventative health care is a key component to good health. It entails testing, medications, and lifestyle choices to prevent disease. Part of preventative health care is healthy living, which includes regular exercise, good nutrition, not smoking, and using alcohol in moderation or not at all.

Review the preventative health care worksheet and note the dates of the previously attained exams. If you are outside the range recommended on the form, discuss with your doctor. See instructions on completing this form in Chapter 7.

STEP FOUR: DIAGNOSTIC TESTING

Every time you have a test, of any kind, get a copy for your personal record. This section can be broken down into four subsections:

- Blood work

- Radiology

- Procedure/Diagnostic Testing

- Surgery

Include blood tests such as complete blood counts, kidney function tests, electrolytes such as potassium and sodium, liver tests, thyroid tests, and cholesterol tests taken in the last five years. It is not necessary to include every lab report. For example, during hospitalization there are often daily blood tests and including each of these will not benefit any health care provider. Also, patients who are on coumadin get blood tests monthly and sometimes more frequently. It is not necessary to include each of these blood tests. Try to obtain the most recent tests of the following:

- Complete blood count

- Kidney test/electrolyte

- Liver function tests

- Thyroid test

- Cholesterol level

There will be many variations based on individual disease profiles.

Radiology reports include X-rays, ultrasounds, CAT scans, MRIs, mammograms, and PET scans. It is not necessary to place the actual film in your record, but do include a copy of your doctor's written report of the interpretation.

Diagnostic tests include a variety of procedures including stress tests, electro-cardiograms, echocardiograms, pap smears, pulmonary function tests, etc. Each test or procedure is accompanied by a written interpretation by the doctor. Include this report in the health care record.

The record should also include a list of all of your procedures. Each procedure that is performed will have a written explanation of the disease. If you have had a diagnostic procedure such as a colonoscopy, endoscopy, angiogram, mammogram, or biopsy, obtain a written copy of the report.

Obtain a copy of any surgical report from your surgeon.

Step 5: Doctor Visits

This is the place to record your health care encounters. This section can be further subdivided into primary care or specialist care visits and hospital/nursing home stays. Each doctor visit can be classified as an acute, follow-up, or mainte-nance (such as an annual exam) visit. Appendix B has a form for each type of visit. The form will allow you to have a good health care encounter and will serve as a record for future reference. See Chapter 4 for more details.

The hospitalization record includes a summary of each hospitalization. Some hospitals provide discharge summaries. If you can get your hands on these sum-maries, they are ideal for your personal record. If you are unable to do so, a form is provided in the appendix that allows you to record vital information about your hospital stay. This serves as an adjunct to the hospital record noted in Section 1.

STEP 6: ADVANCED DIRECTIVES

Advanced directives are wishes that you want carried out in the future. End of life often renders individuals unable to make decisions due to severe illness or mental impairment. Considering many potential options and discussing them with your loved ones and health care provider can help assure that your wishes will be carried out. Everyone should fill out the advanced directive form provided in Appendix A. This form is not a legal document but can help you, your loved ones, and your health care provider understand your wishes regarding end-of-life medical care. This form is a tool to help you start thinking about how you want your medical care to go. The next step is to develop a living will with the help of an attorney to place in your medical record.

DEFINITIONS

ADVANCED DIRECTIVES: Legal statements in which a person may state his or her treatment preferences so they may be honored if the individual becomes incapable of making such decisions.

LIVING WILL: A document that lists interventions that a patient would request, reject, or accept in the future. Usually, this is based on a situation in which one is ill or demented and has no chance of recovering. Some items that need to be addressed are intubations, CPR, dialysis, antibiotic use, artificial means of nutrition, hydration, and surgery. The goal of a living will is to state your wishes in advance of aggressive life-sustaining treatment.

DURABLE POWER OF ATTORNEY FOR HEALTH CARE: A legal document that allows a patient to appoint someone to make decisions if he or she becomes temporarily or permanently incapacitated or is declared incompetent.

DO NOT RESUSCITATE: A statement that says if a person stops breathing or the heart stops, no attempts will be made to resuscitate him or her. It is important to discuss your wishes with your health care provider.

Have him or her explain the process of CPR and make the decision. Make sure that you sign the proper paperwork.

To develop advanced directives, you can go to an attorney (many specialize in elder law) or use software.

Step 7: Chronic Disease

When your health breaks down and chronic disease sets in, managing disease is vital to maintaining function. Partnering with your doctor to manage chronic disease decreases its impact.

All hope is not lost if you become afflicted with a chronic disease. Proper management has the potential to limit the negative effect on your health and function. But it requires that you take health care responsibility.

Chronic disease, defined as disease that persists, affects more than ninety million Americans and accounts for the majority of health care costs and deaths in the United States. The impact of chronic disease will continue to increase as the population ages. Arthritis, heart disease, high blood pressure, stroke, lung disease, Alzheimer's disease, depression, diabetes, and osteoporosis are common chronic disease that leads to death and disability.

Chronic disease is very common in the older population. In those over seventy-five years old, 193 of 1,000 adults have their activity limited by arthritis and other musculoskeletal conditions. Heart and other circulatory conditions is the second most common debilitating condition, limiting activity in 160 of every 1,000 adults over the age of seventy-five, according to the Department of Health and Human Services.

Chronic disease often leads to disability that limits independence. Disability makes it exceedingly difficult for individuals to care for themselves. Activities such as bathing, cooking, eating, dressing, using the toilet, performing housework, managing money, and running errands become more and more as disability increases. It is essential that chronic diseases be managing appropriately to decrease disability.

Personal health care responsibility can have a significant impact on the treatment of chronic disease. This responsibility takes many forms including exercise, good nutrition, avoiding tobacco, and tracking health care.

Management of chronic disease is a partnership between you and your provider, incorporating healthy lifestyle, disease monitoring, and healthcare screenings.

When you are diagnosed with a new disease or condition, do not assume your doctor will take full responsibility in managing it. You are one who has to live with the disease and its impact. The doctor cannot do an adequate job without help from you. Your doctor is like a wide receiver, and you are like the quarterback. Having a good wide receiver can get you a lot of touchdowns but if the quarterback never gets him the ball he will never score. If you do not get the information to your doctor, he or she will never be able to help you. Great quarterbacks can make average receivers look really good.

Section 7 is a place to record information on the chronic diseases. This is the place to store literature on the chronic diseases that afflict you. This book originally described twelve chronic disease and how to personalize the disease. The content became overwhelming and warranted a book of its own. This is fully described in *Health Care Responsibility: Chronic Disease Management (to be released).*

Speak with your doctor about any information that he or she desires for you to collect. Check http://www.hcrbooks.com or the table below for examples of factors that should be tracked in chronic diseases.

TABLE 11-1
SELECTED MONITORING PARAMETERS IN CHRONIC DISEASES

- Diabetes: Blood sugars

- Hypertension: Blood pressure and heart rate readings

- Heart Failure: Daily weights

- Heart Disease and Stroke: Risk factor monitoring

- Incontinence: Voiding diary

SUMMARY

The medical system is a complex, fragmented system. It falls upon the shoulder of each individual to take responsibility for assuring proper health care, which can result in more effective care. Keeping your personal health record updated will help you understand your medical care and make you a partner in the process.

Implementing the personal health care system can result in significant improvements in your health. It helps you communicate effectively in the health care system and prevents you from slipping through the cracks. The payoffs of being an active member of your health care system will be immense.

Start today! Using the knowledge gained in this book, complete the seven steps to your personal health care record. This will start you on the road to health care responsibility. Continue to use the process, and you will be assured the highest quality health care this country has to offer.

SECTION 5

APPENDIXES

APPENDIX A

ESSENTIAL FORMS

Medical Record System

Name: _____

Date of Birth: _____

Sex: _____ Height: _____ Weight/Date recorded: _____

Health Insurance/policy Number: _____

Secondary Health Insurance: _____

Ethnic Background: _____

Religious Affiliation: _____

Highest Level of Education: _____

Living Will: yes/no. Where is it filed? _____

Emergency Contact: _____

Power of Attorney: _____

Occupation: _____

Martial Status: _____ Children: _____

Living Arrangement (alone, spouse, etc.): _____

What type of home do you live in? _____

How many stairs do you have to your front door _____

How many stairs do you have to your 2nd floor _____ basement: _____

Smoking: Yes/No (If applicable) Year Quit: _____ Packs/Day: _____

Years Smoked: _____ Current Tobacco Use: _____

Recreational Drug Use _____

Alcohol Use: Drinks _____ per Day/Week/Month/Year. Date of last drink: _____

Blood Transfusion: Number _____ Dates: _____

Reason: _____

Blood/Rh type: _____

Last Eye Exam: _____ Glasses/Contacts: _____

Last Dental Exam: _____ Dentures: Yes or No

Hearing Aides: Yes or No. Hearing Problems: _____

Immunization Dates

Influenza: _____ Pneumonia: _____ Tetanus/Diphtheria: _____

Drug Allergies   Reaction

_____ - _____

_____ - _____

_____ - _____

_____ - _____

_____ - _____

            - _____

Medical History

_____ _____

_____ _____

_____ _____

_____ _____

_____ _____

_____ _____

_____ _____

_____ _____

_____ _____

Surgeries

_____ _____

_____ _____

_____ _____

_____ _____

_____ _____

Family History

_____

_____

_____

_____

_____

_____

Hospitalizations

_____

_____

_____

_____

_____

_____

Procedures

_____

_____

_____

_____

_____

Doctor List

Doctor Name	Specialty	Phone Number	Address

Medication List

Medication	Dose and Date Started	Time(s) Taken	Reason Taken

Medications Taken in the Past

Medication	Date Started/Stopped	Reason Taken	Reason Stopped	Side Effects/Problems

Daily Medication List

	Monday	Tuesday	Wednesday
Morning			
Noon			
Dinner			
Before Bed			

Thursday	Friday	Saturday	Sunday

Advanced Directives

I, _____, write this health care directive to help my
loved ones and health care providers carry out my wishes.

Durable Power of Attorney for Health Care

_____ I appoint the person listed below to make decisions about my medical care if there comes
a time I am unable to do so myself due to an illness or an advanced dementia. I request that this
person, my health care providers, and family be guided by the decisions I have made as part of
this document.

Name: _____

Address: _____

_____

Phone number: _____

E-mail: _____

If the person above cannot or will not make decisions for me, I appoint this person:

Name: _____

Address: _____

_____

Phone number: _____

E-mail: _____

_____ I have not appointed anyone to make health care decisions for me.

Living Will

If my condition is deemed terminal as indicated below...

Definition of terminal includes (check what applies):

_____ cancer diagnosis with less than _____ months to live

_____ advanced dementia

_____ end stage congestive heart failure

_____ other _____

_____ other _____

...these are my wishes:

I do not want the following life-sustaining treatments.

_____ cardiopulmonary resuscitation

_____ breathing tube

_____ nasogastric tube

_____ intravenous fluid therapy

_____ intravenous antibiotics

_____ oral antibiotics

_____ blood or blood product transfusions

_____ medicines to prolong life that do not aid in my comfort such as cholesterol medicine

_____ artificial nutrition if it would be the main treatment to keep me alive

_____ if artificial treatment is started, I want it stopped

_____ measures to keep me as comfortable as possible, even if they shorten my life.

_____ surgery

_____ other _____

If I am in a persistent vegetative state, I do not want the following life-sustaining treatments.

_____ cardiopulmonary resuscitation
_____ breathing tube
_____ nasogastric tube
_____ intravenous fluid therapy
_____ intravenous antibiotics
_____ oral antibiotics
_____ blood or blood product transfusions
_____ medicines to prolong life that do not aid in my comfort such as cholesterol medicine
_____ artificial nutrition if it would be the main treatment to keep me alive
_____ if artificial treatment is started, I want it stopped
_____ measures to keep me as comfortable as possible, even if they shorten my life
_____ surgery
_____ other _____

Miscellaneous Directions

Many health care situations cannot be foreseen. This section allows health care wishes to be expressed that may be specific to a certain disease state that are not covered under a terminal state or persistent vegetative state.

_____
_____
_____
_____
_____
_____

Organ donation:

_____ I do not want to donate any of my organs or tissues.
_____ I want to donate all of my organs and tissues.
_____ I only want to donate these organs and tissues:

_____

Autopsy

_____ I do not want an autopsy
_____ I agree to an autopsy if it is my health care provider's wish
_____ I want an autopsy, regardless whether my health care provider wishes
_____ other wishes

_____

Any other wishes

_____
_____
_____
_____
_____
_____
_____
_____
_____

_____
_____
_____
_____
_____
_____
_____
_____
_____
_____
_____
_____
_____
_____
_____
_____
_____
_____
_____

Signature

Your signature must accompany the signature of two witnesses

Signature: _____

Date: _____

Address: _____

Witness

I believe that the person who signed above to be in sound mind and this document was signed in my presence. This advanced directive was not filled out or signed under pressure, fraud, or undue influence.

I meet no criteria listed below:

- Related to by marriage, blood, or adoption to the person making this advanced directive
- The person appointed in this advanced directive
- The health care provider or an employee of the provider responsible for the person in this advanced directive.

Signature: _____

Print name: _____

Date: _____

Address: _____

Signature: _____

Print name: _____

Date: _____

Address: _____

Health Evaluation Worksheet for Healthy Males and Females over age 50

Date						
	Recommendation	Results	Results	Results	Results	Follow-up/comments
Exams						
Physical exam	Annual					
Breast exam (female)	Annual					
Pelvic exam/Pap (female)	1-3 years					
Prostate evaluation (male)	Annual at age 40-50					
Dental exam	Every 6 months					
Eye exam	1-3 years					
Hearing screen	Annual					
Diagnostic Tests						
Blood pressure	Every two years					
Mammography (female)	Annual					
DEXA (female)	At age 65					
Blood in the stool	Annual after 50					
Sigmoidoscopy	Every 5 years (at 50)					
Colonoscopy	Every 10 years (at50)					
Abdominal ultrasound	once in smokers					
Ankle-brachial index	At 70, high risk at 50					
Tuberculosis	High-risk people					
EKG	Once					
Chest X-ray	None					
Blood Test						
Blood count (CBC)	1-5 years					
Thyroid test	1-5 years					
Kidney function	1-5 years					
Diabetes screen	High-risk people					
Cholesterol	1-5 years					
PSA (men)	every year over 50					
Screens						
Skin	Annual					
Depression	Annual					
Dementia	Annual					
Medication review	Annual					
Obesity	Annual					
Immunizations						
Influenza	Annual					
Pneumonia	At age 65					
Tetanus/Diphtheria	Every 10 years					
Counseling						
Exercise	Annual					
Diet	Annual					
Smoking/Tobacco	Annual					
Alcohol	Annual					

APPENDIX B

ENCOUNTER FORMS

There are three main types of doctor's appointments: acute visits, maintenance evaluations, and follow-up appointments. The acute visit is used when the patient has a medical problem such as a cough or fever and needs an immediate evaluation. Maintenance visits do not require urgency and can be set up at the convenience of the doctor and the patient. The annual physical exam is an example. Follow-up visits are used when the health care provider needs to evaluate the effectiveness of a treatment or monitor a chronic disease. For example, when a patient is started on a new blood pressure medicine, the doctor will schedule a follow-up visit to evaluate the effectiveness and any negative consequences of the drug.

The acute visit form will help you organize information when presenting with a new health care issue. It includes a section to record instructions on treatment and follow-up. The form is set up to become part of your health record.

These steps will help you fill out the acute visit form.

1. Record the doctor's name, the date, and a brief description of the problems.

2. Describe your specific symptoms. See acute visit describing information in this appendix for information that will help your doctor determine the origin of your problem.

3. Bring the form to your appointment and record the doctor's diagnosis.

4. Record the names of any medications that the doctor prescribes and ask a) how to take it/how long to take it, b) side effects, and c) any follow-up required.

5. Record any other treatments ordered.

6. Record any testing the doctor wants performed, including radiology or laboratory work.

7. Most importantly, record what type of follow-up is necessary. It is important to specifically ask when you should be seen back in the office, when to call the office, and what information you can gather about this problem that will help your evaluation. For example, daily weights

are helpful in evaluating response to treatment of congestive heart failure to record weight fluctuations.

The follow-up visit form helps you relay information to the doctor after a specific problem has been diagnosed. It is a place for you to record information that the doctor needs to track how your disease is progressing or how you are responding to treatment. This section may include a variety of things. Many things being evaluated for may be better tracked with specific chronic disease forms. For more information, see http://www.hcrbooks.com. Anytime you are seen for an acute visit, you should ask, "What information can I gather about this problem that will help your evaluation?" This form is a place to gather that information.

Patients who are diagnosed with diabetes will need frequent follow-up visits. Monitoring blood sugars and blood pressure will help your doctor. There will be situations when a more general form will be useful; one example would be if a patient has a fever and the doctor is not sure where that fever is coming form. The follow-up form can be a place where the patient can record dates and times of his or her temperature and any other symptoms.

Use the annual form to record information that will help your doctor give you a comprehensive evaluation. In the first section, list any changes in the last year including medical illness, surgeries, exercise, alcohol consumption, and smoking. The form includes a section to record any symptoms. Social functioning is important to the overall health of the older patient. The annual form includes some questions that will help the doctor screen you for depression. It also provides a list of activities and asks you to rate how well you are functioning with these specific tasks. Activities include feeding, toileting, dressing, and bathing, to name a few. The form concludes with a list of questions that you should ask your care provider to ensure he or she is evaluating all aspects of good preventative health care. Bring along the preventative health care worksheet and go through each item on the list. Reviewing the guidelines provided in Chapter 5 will help you understand what testing should be done.

The last form is the question form to record a list of questions you want your health care provider to answer. Report the questions in order of importance. Realize that you may not get to ask all your questions during the office visit. Make one copy for you and one for your health care provider.

Acute Visit Form

Doctor seen: _____ Date:_____

Reason for visit: _____

Symptom   Describing information

_____   _____
                         _____
                         _____
                         _____
_____   _____
                         _____
                         _____
                         _____
_____   _____
                         _____
                         _____
                         _____

Diagnosis: _____

Treatment Ordered

Medicine name: _____
How to take it: _____
Side effects: _____
How to follow up: _____
Medicine name: _____
How to take it: _____
Side effects: _____
How to follow up: _____
Medicine name: _____
How to take it: _____
Side effects: _____
How to follow up: _____
Other Treatments: _____
_____

Recommended Testing: _____
_____

Follow-up:
When should I be seen back in the office? _____
Under what circumstances should I call you? _____
_____

What type of information can I gather to help you with your evaluation? _____
_____
_____
_____

Acute visit describing information

Abdominal pain
When did it start?
Where is the pain located? Is it located all over the stomach or is the pain localized in one area of the stomach? Has the location of pain changed over the course of the pain?
How long has the pain lasted? Is the pain constant or does it come and go?
What is the pain like? Dull, sharp, burning, etc.?
Any other symptoms—nausea, vomiting, poor appetite, fever, chills, or heartburn?
Does the pain radiate anywhere else?
Is the pain worse at any given time such as after meals or in the morning? Does anything make it better, such as having a bowel movement or sleeping?
How bad is the pain on a scale of 0-10 with 0 being no pain and 10 being the most severe you can imagine?

Back pain
When did it start?
Where is it located?
How long has the pain lasted? Is it constant or does it come and go?
What is the pain like? Dull, sharp, burning, etc.?
Any other symptoms? Any changes with urination or bowel movements? Do you have a fever?
Does the pain radiate anywhere else?
What makes the pain worse or better?
How bad is the pain on a scale of 0-10 with 0 being no pain and 10 being the most severe you can imagine?

Cough
When did it start?
Is the cough dry or moist?
Is the cough productive or nonproductive? What time of day is it worst? What is the color of the sputum? Does the color clear as the day progresses? Is the mucous thick or thin?
Is there any wheezing?
Is there any shortness of breath, fever, chills, poor appetite, fever, wheeze, chest pain, or burning in the chest?
Are you short of breath when you are lying down?

Chest pain
When did it start?
Where is it located?
How long has it lasted?
Describe the pain. Is it sharp, stabbing, aching, or feel like pressure etc.?
Are you having any other symptoms such as shortness of breath, nausea, or sweating?
Does the pain radiate? Where?
Does movement make the pain worse?
How bad is the pain on a scale of 0-10 with 0 being no pain and 10 being the most severe you can imagine?

Constipation
When did it start?
How often do you have bowel movements?
Is the stool hard?
Do you have abdominal pain?
Any changes in medicines?
How much fluid do you drink?

Diarrhea
When did it start?
How many times a day do you have diarrhea?
Do you notice diarrhea after eating certain foods?
Do you have diarrhea at night?
Do you have any abdominal pain?
Do you have a fever?
Have you had any changes in your diet?
Have you traveled recently?

Dizziness
When did it start?
Describe the dizziness. Does it feel like the room is spinning? Do you feel like you are going to pass out? Do you feel unsteady when you walk?
Have you had any loss of consciousness?
Have you any chest pain, shortness of breath, visual changes, hearing changes, or ringing in the ears?

Edema/Swelling
When did it start?
Where is the swelling?
Do you have a fever or chills?
Do you have any shortness of breath when lying down?
Any skin changes, such as redness?
Do you have any shortness of breath or chest pain?
Any changes in your urination?
Any changes in your appetite?

Fatigue
When did it start?
What makes it worse or better?
Have you had any weakness?
Have you had any fever?
Are you depressed?
Has your eating habits changed?
Any weight loss?
Any pain?

Have there been any changes in your sleep patterns?

Headache
When did it start?
Where is it located?
How long has the pain lasted? Is it constant or does it come and go?
Describe the pain—is it sharp or dull or does it cause numbness?
What makes the pain worse or better?
How bad is the pain on a scale of 0-10 with 0 being no pain and 10 being the most severe you can imagine?
Any other symptoms such as nausea, vomiting, neck pain, dizziness, numbness, visual changes, eye tearing, or nasal congestion?

Joint Pain
When did it start?
Where is it located?
How long has the pain lasted? Is it constant or does it come and go?
Describe the pain—is it sharp or dull or does it cause numbness?
Does the pain radiate? Where?
What makes the pain worse or better?
How bad is the pain on a scale of 0-10 with 0 being no pain and 10 being the most severe you can image?
Any other symptoms or any changes with urination or bowel movements or a fever?

Nausea
When did it start?
Have you vomited?
Do you have any other symptoms? Pain, sweating, diarrhea, constipation, etc.?
Have you taken any new medicines?

Runny nose
When did it start?
Describe the discharge: thin or thick? A small, medium, or large amount?
Any other symptoms such as cough, sore throat, earache, fever, headache, or body aches?

Shortness of breath
When did it start?
When does it occur? For example, during exertion or when lying down at night.
Do you have any chest pain or leg swelling?
Have you been coughing?

Sore throat
When did it start?
Any other symptoms such as fever, runny nose, cough, or eye discharge?
Any change in your appetite?

Urinary incontinence
When did it start?
Do you need to urinate urgently?
Do you leak after you void?
Do you urinate frequently at night?
How many times a day to you urinate?
Do you have any burning with urination?
How much do you leak?
Have you birthed any children? Vaginally? C-section?
Do you have any genital itching/discharge/rash/pain?
How long can you hold urine after you feel the urge?
Do you need to strain to void?
What color is the urine? Is there a strong odor?

Annual Form

Have you had any major illnesses or surgeries in the past year? _____

_____

_____

_____

Have you had any new illness or deaths in your family over the last year? _____

_____

_____

_____

How much have you been…

exercising: _____

smoking: _____

using alcohol: _____

Circle all symptoms you have had over the last three months. Describe in detail any symptom listed below.

General	Sensory	Head & Neck	Chest/Lungs	Genital/Urinary	Stomach	Muscle & Skeleton	Psychiatric
Fatigue	Vision changes	Runny nose	Chest pain, tightness or pressure	Burning on urination	Nausea	Joint pain	Depression
Weight loss	Double vision	Nasal congestion	Shortness of breath	Urinary frequency	Vomiting	Stiffness	Anxiety
Weight gain	Blurred vision	Sore throat	Difficulty breathing when lying down	Urinary urgency	Diarrhea	Swelling	Hallucinations
Not hungry	Decreased hearing	Headache	Cough	Urinary hesitancy	Constipation	Weakness	Delusions
Difficulty sleeping	Numbness	Tooth pain	Coughing up blood	Blood in urine	Blood in stool		Memory loss
Falls	Tingling	Facial pain	Shortness of breath on exertion	A lot of urinating at night	Change in appetite		Confusion
Skin problems	Dizziness	Difficulty chewing	Palpitations or irregular heart beat	Urinary Incontinence			
	Headache	Difficulty Swallowing					

Men	Women
Pain or lumps in your testicles	Breast changes
Any sexual dysfunction/ability to get or maintain an erection	Menstrual changes
	Vaginal discharge or bleeding
	Pain with intercourse

Describe in detail any symptoms circled above:

_____
_____
_____
_____
_____
_____
_____
_____
_____

Social Questions:

1. Have you had any changes in your living arrangement?   Y   N
2. Have you had any change in relationships?   Y   N
3. Have you had any changes in your finances?   Y   N
4. Have you had a decreased ability to perform activities of daily living?   Y   N

Describe: _____
_____
_____

Depression Screen

1. Do you feel depressed, sad, or blue?   Y   N
2. Have you lost interest in many activities you previously enjoyed?   Y   N
3. Do you have problems sleeping?   Y   N
4. Do you suffer from lack of energy?   Y   N
5. Are you frequently unable to concentrate?   Y   N
6. Have you had any appetite change?   Y   N
7. Do you frequently feel irritable, restless, anxious, or withdrawn?   Y   N
8. Do you feel bad about yourself or have a lot of guilt?   Y   N
9. Do you think things would be easier if you were dead?   Y   N
10. Do you ever think about killing yourself?   Y   N

Describe: _____
_____
_____
_____

Check the column that best describes your ability to do the following activities.

	Independent	Some help	Heavy assistance	Complete Dependence
Bathing				
Toileting				
Walking				
Dressing				
Grooming				
Feeding				
Managing money				
Handyman work				
Taking Medications				
Getting around town				
Laundry				
Housekeeping				
Meals				
Shopping				
Using the telephone				

Questions to ask your health care provider
1. Are all of my medicines necessary?
2. Do I need any routine lab work such as blood counts, kidney function, diabetes tests, cholesterol tests, or thyroid tests? (Refer to the preventative health care worksheet.)
3. Do I need any diagnostic tests such as a mammogram, tests for colon cancer, EKG, bone density tests? (Refer to the preventative health care worksheet.)
4. Are there any unusually findings on my exam?
5. Do I need a pelvic, breast, or prostate exam?
6. Did you screen me for depression and dementia?
7. Do I need any vaccinations such as tetanus, pneumonia, or flu?
8. Can you give me any advice about lifestyle modifications that will make me healthier?

Follow-up Form

Problem being seen for: _____

Information being tracked: _____

_____

_____

_____

_____

_____

_____

_____

_____

_____

_____

_____

_____

_____

_____

_____

_____

_____

_____

_____

_____

_____

_____

_____

_____

_____

_____

_____

_____

Question Form

Record, in order of importance, the questions you want your health care provider to answer. The most important question that you want answered should be number one. Realize that you may not get to ask all of your questions during the office visit. Make one copy for you and one for your provider.

1. _____
   _____
   _____
2. _____
   _____
   _____
3. _____
   _____
   _____
4. _____
   _____
   _____
5. _____
   _____
   _____
6. _____
   _____
   _____
7. _____
   _____
   _____
8. _____
   _____
   _____
9. _____
   _____
   _____
10. _____
    _____
    _____

Hospital Form

Primary Doctor: _____

Phone number: _____ Times rounding: _____

Specialty Doctor: _____

Phone number: _____ Times rounding: _____

Specialty Doctor: _____

Phone number: _____ Times rounding: _____

Specialty Doctor: _____

Phone number: _____ Times rounding: _____

Charge Nurse: _____

Phone number: _____ Available: _____

Date	Doctor	Tests/Labs/Notes

Medicine and dose	Time(s)											

New medicine	Why

New diagnosis

_____
_____
_____
_____

Labs

_____
_____
_____
_____

Diagnostic tests

_____
_____
_____
_____

Surgeries/Procedures

_____
_____
_____
_____
_____

List of Questions

_____
_____
_____
_____
_____
_____
_____
_____
_____
_____
_____
_____
_____
_____
_____
_____

Questions you should ask every day:
1. Is my condition improving or worsening?
2. What is my diagnosis/Have you made any new diagnoses?
3. Have you changed any medicines?
4. Any new treatments other than medicines?
5. How are my laboratory or other test results?
6. What new tests (blood, X-ray, CAT scan etc.) will be done today or tomorrow?
7. Do you have an anticipated discharge date?

Notes

_____
_____
_____
_____
_____
_____
_____
_____
_____
_____
_____
_____
_____

Nursing Home Form

Name:_____

Reason for being at the nursing home:

_____

Doctor's name: _____

Doctor's phone number: _____

Charge nurse: _____

Physical therapist: _____

Occupational therapist: _____

Speech therapist: _____

Physical therapy rehabilitation plan of care:

_____

_____

_____

Occupational therapy rehabilitation plan of care:

_____

_____

_____

Speech therapy rehabilitation plan of care:

_____

Follow-up doctor appointments/Purpose of the visit:

_____

_____

_____

Follow-up tests (X-ray, laboratory):

_____

_____

_____

New treatments/medications:

_____

_____

_____

Anticipated discharge date:

_____

Referral Form

Patient: _____

Primary doctor_____

Primary doctor phone number: _____

Reason for the referral:

_____

_____

_____

_____

_____

Testing already performed, including lab work and diagnostic tests (attach copies):

_____

_____

_____

_____

_____

_____

_____

_____

_____

_____

_____

Recommendations of the specialist (or attach progress note):

_____

_____

_____

_____

_____

_____

_____

_____

_____

_____

_____

_____

_____

_____

_____

Emergency Room Form

Patient: _____

ER and doctor names: _____

Reason for the ER visit:

_____
_____
_____

Testing performed in the ER (attach copies if possible):

_____
_____
_____

Diagnosis in ER:

_____
_____

Treatment in ER:

_____
_____
_____
_____
_____
_____

Discharge instructions:

_____
_____
_____
_____
_____
_____
_____

Follow-up with primary doctor/specialist:

_____
_____
_____
_____
_____
_____

Wash

Your

Hands

HEALTH CARE RESPONSIBILITY

SELECTED REFERENCES

Chapter 2

[1]World Health Organization. "World Health Organization Assesses the World's Health Systems." http://www.who.int/inf-pr-2000/en/pr2000-44.html. Accessed July 13, 2006.

[2]Center of Medicare or Medicaid Services National Health Expenditure Data. http://www.cms.hhs.gov/NationalHealthExpendData/ 02_NationalHealthAccountsHistorical.asp#TopOfPage. Accessed June 21, 2006.

[3]Center for American Progress. "48.4 million and counting." http:// www.americanprogress.org/site/pp.asp?c=biJRJ8OVF&b=1010201. Accessed July 13, 2006.

[4]Center of Disease Control. "Nursing Home Care." http://www.cdc.gov/nchs/ fastats/nursingh.htrn. Accessed July 16, 2006.

[5]Lazarou, J., B. H. Pomeranz, and P. N. Correy. "Incidence of adverse drug reactions: a meta-analysis of prospective studies." *Journal of the American Medical Association,* 279, No. 15 (April 15, 1998), pp. 1200-5.

[6]Institute of Medicine. Insuring Americans Health. Principles and Recommendations. http://www.iom.edu/?id=17632&redirect=0. Accessed June 21, 2006.

Chapter 3

[1]Administration on Aging. Statistics on the Aging Population. http://www.aoa.gov/prof/Statistics/statistics.asp. Accessed July 14, 2006.

[2]Centers of Disease Control. Life Expectancy. http://www.cdc.gov/nchs/fastats/lifexpec.htrn. Accessed July 13, 2006.

Chapter 5

[1]Kohn, L. T., J. M. Corrigan, and M. S. Donaldson. To Err is Human: building a safer health system. Institute of Medicine: National Academy Press, 2000.

[2]Center for Disease Control. Public Health Focus: surveillance, prevention and control of nosocomial infections. MMWR 1992; 41:783-787.

Chapter 7

[1]Merck Manual of Geriatrics. Clinical Pharmacology. http://www.merck.com/mrkshared/mmg/sec1/ch6/ch6a.jsp. Accessed July 14, 2006.

[2]Lazarou, J., B. H. Pomeranz, and P. N. Corey. "Incidence of adverse drug reactions in hospitalized patients: a meta-analysis of prospective studies. *"Journal of the American Medical Association,* 279, No. 15 (April 15, 1998), pp. 1200-5.

[3]Lyles, Alan. "Direct Marketing of Pharmaceuticals to Consumers." *Annual Review of Public Health,* 23, No. 1 (2002), p. 73.

[4]Lesser, K. E., P. D. Allen, S. J. Woolhandler, D. U. Himmelstein, S. M. Wolfe, and D. H. Bor. "Timing of new black box warnings and withdrawals for prescription medications." *Journal of the American Medical Association,* 287, No. 17 (May 1, 2002), pp. 2215-20.